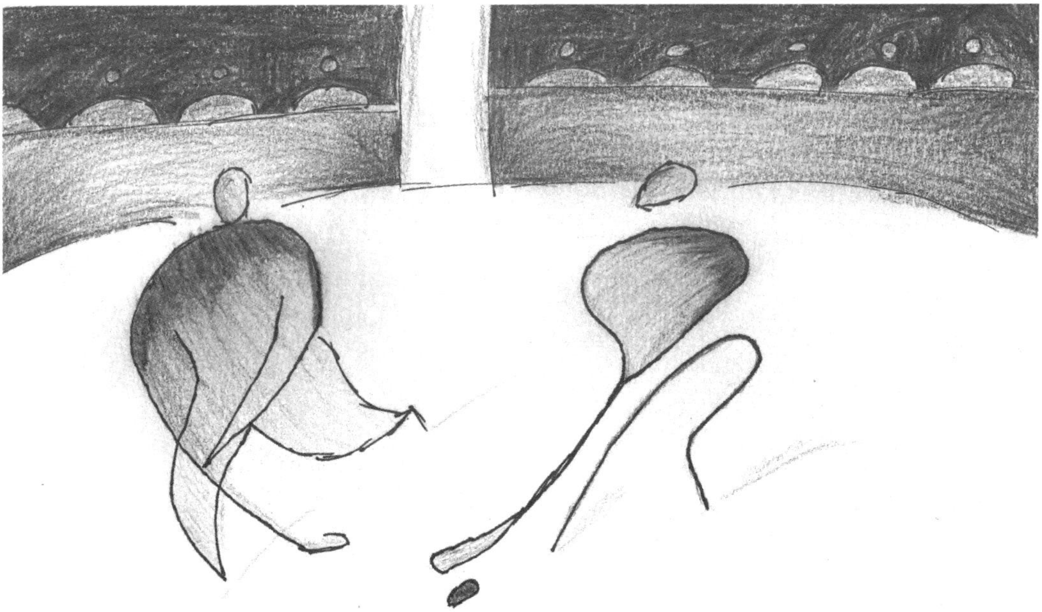

ᒑᓂᑲᓐ ᓚᓐᑎᓐ ᐅᑎᐹᒋᒧᐧᐃᓐ ᒥᔅᑎᓯᓃᐦᒡ ᐅᐦᒋᐤ

ᐧᒑᓇᓓᓐ ᓚᓐᑕᓐ ᐅᑎᐹᒋᒧᐧᐃᓐ, ᒥᔅᑎᓯᓃᐅᐄᓈ

L'histoire de Jonathan Linton de Mistissini

The Story of Jonathan Linton of Mistissini

Told by Jonathan Linton

Written by Ruth DyckFehderau

Translated into Northern East Cree by Luci Bobbish-Salt

Translated into Southern East Cree by Louise Blacksmith

Translated into French by Valérie Duro

ᒥᔪᐱᒫᑎᓰᐅᓐ ᐊᓈᓈᑭᒋᐦᑖᑭᓈᒡ

CONSEIL CRI DE LA SANTÉ ET DES SERVICES SOCIAUX DE LA BAIE JAMES

CREE BOARD OF HEALTH AND SOCIAL SERVICES OF JAMES BAY

Funding for this publication was provided in part by Health Canada. The opinions expressed in this publication are those of the storyteller and do not necessarily reflect the official views of Health Canada or of the Cree Board of Health and Social Services of James Bay.

First printing, 2020. Printed and bound in Canada by Houghton Boston Printers, Saskatoon, Saskatchewan. Distributed by Wilfrid Laurier University Press / wlupress.wlu.ca

Set in Verdana font, chosen for its readability. Printed on paper that is Forest Stewardship Council-certified with post-consumer recycled fibres, and that is acid- and chlorine-free.

Cover design by Nicole Ritzer, based on an original design by Cameron Mosimann. Photograph of Mistissini burnt forest (reversed) taken by David DyckFehderau.

Title page illustration by Semera Coon of Mikw Chiyâm Arts Concentration Program, Voyageur Memorial High School, Mistissini, QC.

Published by Cree Board of Health and Social Services of James Bay
Contact: Paul Linton, 168 Main St, Mistissini, QC, Canada, G0W 1C0 / (418) 923-3355
creehealth.org / sweetbloods.org

Library and Archives Canada Cataloguing in Publication

Title: Chaanithin lintin utipaachimuwin mistisiniihch uhchiiu = Chaanathan lintan utipaachimuwin, mistisiniiuiinuu = L'histoire de Jonathan Linton de Mistissini = The story of Jonathan Linton of Mistissini / story by Jonathan Linton ; translator Northern East Cree, Luci Bobbish-Salt ; translator Southern East Cree, Louise Blacksmith ; translator French Valérie Duro ; writer, Ruth DyckFehderau.

Other titles: Chaanathan lintan utipaachimuwin, mistisiniiuiinuu | Histoire de Jonathan Linton de Mistissini | Story of Jonathan Linton of Mistissini

Names: DyckFehderau, Ruth, author. | DyckFehderau, Ruth, 1967- Story of Jonathan Linton of Mistissini. | DyckFehderau, Ruth, 1967- Story of Jonathan Linton of Mistissini. Cree. | DyckFehderau, Ruth, 1967- Story of Jonathan Linton of Mistissini. French. | Cree Board of Health and Social Services of James Bay, issuing body.

Description: Cree title romanized. | "This is a four-language translation of a single story from The Sweet Bloods of Eeyou Istchee: Stories of Diabetes and the James Bay Cree. (Sweet Bloods contains 26 stories.)" | Text in Northern East Cree, Southern East Cree, French, and English.

Identifiers: Canadiana 20200402889E | ISBN 9781989796023 (softcover)

Subjects: LCSH: Linton, Jonathan (Of Mistissini)—Health. | LCSH: Diabetics—Cree Nation of Mistissini—Biography. | LCGFT: Biographies.

Classification: LCC RC660 .D93 2020 | DDC 362.1964/620092—dc23

Catalogage avant publication de Bibliothèque et Archives Canada

Titre: Chaanithin lintin utipaachimuwin mistisiniihch uhchiiu = Chaanathan lintan utipaachimuwin, mistisiniiuiinuu = L'histoire de Jonathan Linton de Mistissini = The story of Jonathan Linton of Mistissini / story by Jonathan Linton ; translator Northern East Cree, Luci Bobbish-Salt ; translator Southern East Cree, Louise Blacksmith ; translator French Valérie Duro ; writer, Ruth DyckFehderau.

Autres titres: Chaanathan lintan utipaachimuwin, mistisiniiuiinuu | Histoire de Jonathan Linton de Mistissini | Story of Jonathan Linton of Mistissini

Noms: DyckFehderau, Ruth, 1967- auteur. | DyckFehderau, Ruth, 1967- Story of Jonathan Linton of Mistissini. | DyckFehderau, Ruth, 1967- Story of Jonathan Linton of Mistissini. Cree. | DyckFehderau, Ruth, 1967- Story of Jonathan Linton of Mistissini. Français. | Conseil Cri de la santé et des services sociaux de la Baie-James, organisme de publication.

Description: Titre cri romanisé. | Histoire publiée antérieurement dans : The Sweet Bloods of Eeyou Istchee: Stories of Diabetes and the James Bay Cree. | Texte en cri de l'Est du nord, en cri de l'Est du sud, en français et en anglais.

Identifiants: Canadiana 20200402889F | ISBN 9781989796023 (couverture souple)

Vedettes-matière: RVM: Linton, Jonathan—Santé. | RVM: Diabétiques—Cree Nation of Mistissini—Biographies. | RVMGF: Biographies.

Classification: LCC RC660 .D93 2020 | CDD 362.1964/620092—dc23

ᐧᒑᓂᓕᓐ ᑳᐹᑦ ᐊᓂᑎᐦ ᐅᐦᒋ ᐅᑖᐹᓈᔅᑯᐦᒡ,
ᓈᑖᐦ ᓃᐱᓰᐦᒡ ᐋᑐᐦᑖᑦ, ᐊᓂᑖᐦ ᐋᔑ ᓯᒋᑦ
ᑰᓂᐦᒡ, ᒫᐧᑳᒡ ᐧᐄᔖᑯᐲᓯᒻᐦ ᒌᐦ ᐊᑯᒋᓂᔨᐤᐦ
ᑳ ᓂᑐᐦᐅᒡ ᐅᐦᑖᐧᐄᐦ᙮ ᑳ ᒌᔑ ᓯᒋᑦ ᒦᓐ
ᐊᓂᑖᐦ ᐋᔑ ᐴᓯᑦ ᐅᑖᐹᓈᔅᑯᐦᒡ, ᒦᓐ ᐋᑎ
ᒋᔥᒋᐱᔨᔨᒡᐦ ᐅᐦᑖᐧᐄᐦ᙮ ᐹᐦᑳᒡ ᒌᐦ ᐱᒥᐱᔨᔪᐧᐃᒡ
ᐋᐦ ᓈᓂᑎᐧᐋᐱᐦᑎᐦᒡ ᐋᐦ ᐋᑎᔅᒋᔨᒡᐦ ᐊᐧᐋᔨᐤᐦ,
ᑳᐦ ᐱᒧᐦᑖᔨᐧᑳᓂᐦᐄ ᑳᒄᐦ ᑭᔮᐦ ᒫᒃ ᐱᔮᐤᐦ᙮
ᒋᐱᐦᒌᐦ ᒥᐧᔮᔨᐦᑎᒧᒡ ᒌᐦ ᐧᐋᐱᐦᑖᒡ ᒨᔅᐦ᙮ ᐋᔥᒄ
ᓂᒥᓂᐦᑖᐦ ᐅᐦᒋ ᒌᐦ ᐹᔅᒋᐧᓵᐤ ᐧᒑᓂᓕᓐ ᒨᔅᐦ᙮
ᐃᔮᐹᐦᒃ ᓂᐱᔨᐤ ᑭᔮᐦ ᒫᓂᐦᐧᑳᑦ᙮ ᓈᔥᒡ ᐋᐦ
ᑯᔥᐧᑳᔨᐦᑎᐦᒃ ᓈᔥᒡ ᐋᐦ ᐹᔥᑖᔨᒡ ᐲᐦᒡ ᐅᑐᓐ᙮
ᐅᔮ ᐋᔥᐱᐦᒑᒋᔖᐹᔭᔨᒡ ᓃᔕ ᓂᔅᑲᐦ ᒌᐦ
ᓂᐱᐦᐋᐧᐃᒡ ᑭᔮᐦ ᐊᓂᑖᐦ ᐅᑖᐦᒡ ᐅᑖᐹᓈᔅᑯᐦᒡ
ᐋᑯᑖᐦ ᑳᐦ ᐋᐱᔨᒡᐦ ᐊᓂᔮᐦ ᓂᔅᑲᐦ᙮ ᒦᓐ ᐹᐦᑳᒡ
ᐋᑎ ᐱᒥᐱᔨᒡ᙮

ᒥᒄ ᒫᒃ = ᒦᓐ ᐧᐄᐦ ᓯᒋᐤ ᐧᒑᓂᓕᓐ᙮ ᒦᓐ᙮
ᒑᐱᐦᒋᔨᒡᐦ ᐅᐦᑖᐧᐄᐦ᙮

ᐧᐋᓴ, ᓂᐧᐃᒡ ᐋᓯᐦᒡ ᒋᐱᐦᒌᐧᐃᒡ᙮

ᓂᔮᓈᓈᐤ ᑎᐦᐧᑖᐤ ᒌᐦ ᒋᓯᐤ ᐊᓂᔮ ᒥᒄ ᐹᔨᐧᑳᐤ
ᐋᐦ ᒌᓂᐧᑳᓂᐦᑖᔨᒡᐦ ᐲᓯᒧᐦᑳᓐᐦ᙮ ᑖᓂᑖᐦ ᐧᐋᐦᒋ
ᓇᔥᒡ ᒌᐦ ᒥᐦᒫᑭᒥᔨᒡ ᐊᐧᐋᓐ ᓂᐲᔨᐤ ᐲᐦᒡ ᐋᐦ
ᐄᐦᑖᑦ᙮ ᒫᐧᑳᔨᐤ ᒫ ᐅᐦᒋ ᒋᔨᐱᑖᑦ ᐅᐲᒌᓯᒻᐦ
ᐧᐋᔥ ᐧᐄᐱᒡ ᒦᓐ ᑭᑎ ᐧᐄᐦ ᓯᒋᐤ᙮ ᑭᔮᐦ ᒫᒃ
ᐅᔮ ᐅᑐᓐ ᑖᓐ ᐋᓂᔨᒡ ᓈᔥᒡ ᐋᐦ ᐹᔥᑖᔨᒡ᙮
ᑭᔮᐦ ᐊᑐᒡ ᐅᐦᒋ ᓂᐲᐅᔨᐤ ᒥᓯᓂᐦᐄᑭᓈᒋᓂᔨᐤ
ᒌᐦ ᑎᑯᐦᑎᐦᒃ ᑳ ᐄᔥᐱᔑ ᐹᔥᑖᔨᒡ ᐊᓂᔮ
ᐅᑐᓐ᙮ ᐋᑳᔮᐱᑖᔨᐦᑦ ᑯᑎᒡ ᒫᐧᑳᓐ, ᐄᑏᓯ

ᒌ ᐧᐄᐧᐄᐤ ᐧᒑᓇᓓᓐ ᐊᓂᔫ ᐴᔥᑖᓰᑖᐸᓂᔫ,
ᒥᔅᑎᑯᔅᑳᐦᒡ ᑳ ᐃᔑ ᒋᔅᑐᐦᑌᑦ ᒉ ᓂᑑ ᓯᒋᑦ᙮
ᓵᔅ ᒌ ᑰᓅᓂᔫ᙮ ᐊᑎᐦᑲᒣᑯᐲᓯᒻ ᒌ ᐊᑯᒋᓅ᙮
ᑳ ᒌᔑᐊᐃᐦᑎᑦ ᐁᒄ ᒦᓐ ᑳ ᐴᓯᑦ ᐊᓂᔫ
ᐅᑖᐹᓂᔫ ᐁᒄ ᒦᓐ ᑳ ᒋᐦᒋᐸᔨᐧᑖᐤ ᐊᓂᔫᐦ
ᐅᐦᑖᐧᐄᐦ ᐁ ᐱᒥᐸᔨᐦᑖᔨᒡ᙮ ᐯᐦᑳᒡ ᒌ ᐊᑎ
ᐱᒥᐸᔫᒡ ᐁ ᐊᐃᑖᐱᐧᑖᐤ ᐊᓂᑌ ᐧᐄᐧᐄᑎᒥᐦᒡ
ᐁ ᓈᓂᑑᐧᐁᔨᐦᑕᐦᐧᑳᐤ ᐧᐃᔦᔅ ᒉᒌ ᐁᑕᔅᒋᔨᒡ
ᐊᐧᐁᓰᔅ ᒧᐧᐁᐦᒡ ᑳᒄ ᒫᒃ ᐱᔦᐤᐦ᙮ ᓄᐧᐊᒡ ᒋᐹ
ᒨᒋᑲᓐ ᒫᑖᐦᐋᐧᑖᐤ ᒨᓯ᙮ ᐁᔅᒄ ᓇᒧᐃ ᐅᐦᒋ
ᓂᐸᐦᐁᐤ ᐧᒑᓇᓓᓐ ᒨᓯ᙮ ᑳ ᐅᑎᓇᐦᒃ ᐴᑖᔫ
ᓂᐱᔫ ᐁ ᐃᐦᑕᑯᓂᔨᒡ ᐊᓂᑕ ᑳ ᐋᐸᐦᐊᐦᒃ
ᐁᒄ ᑳ ᐧᑳᔥᑕᑯᒧᑦ ᐊᓂᔫ ᓂᐱᔫ᙮ ᑖᐧᐯ ᒌ
ᐹᐦᑯᑖᐦᑕᒧᑯᐸᓄ ᐁᑳ ᐅᐦᒋ ᒋᔅᒉᔨᐦᑕᐦᒃ᙮
ᒌ ᓂᐸᐦᑖᑌᐅᒡ ᐊᓂᔫ ᑳ ᒉᒋᒐᐹᔭᔨᒡ,
ᐊᓂᑌ ᐅᑖᐦᒡ ᐅᑖᐹᓂᒡ ᐁᑯᑦ ᑳ ᐊᐦᐋᐧᑖᐤ
ᓃᔕ ᓂᔅᑲᐦ᙮ ᐧᐁᐧᐁᔨᑦ ᒌ ᐱᒥᐸᔫᒡ ᐊᓂᔫ
ᐯᒥᐸᔨᐧᑖᐤ᙮

ᓇᒧᐃ ᒋᓄᐅᔥ ᓵᔅ ᒦᓐ ᐧᐋᐦ ᓯᒋᑦ᙮ ᐁᒄ ᑮᐹ ᑳ
ᒋᐱᐦᒋᐸᔨᐦᑖᔨᒡ ᐅᐦᑖᐧᐄ ᐊᓂᔫ ᐅᑖᐸᓂᔫ᙮

ᐊᑕᒫ ᑖᐧᐯ᙮

ᓵᔅ ᓂᔮᐃᐧᓈᐤ ᒌ ᓯᒎ ᐯᔭᐧᑳᐤ ᐁ ᒌᓂᐧᑳᓂᐦᑌᔨᒡ
ᐧᐊᒡ᙮ ᐊᑕᒫᑖᐧᐯᐦ᙮ ᓇᒧᐃ ᒉᒋᒻ ᒋᓄᐅᔥ ᑳ
ᒋᐳᐱᑖᑦ ᐅᐸᐃᒌᓯᒻᐦ ᓵᔅ ᒦᓐ ᐧᐋ ᓯᒋᑦ, ᑖᓐ
ᐧᐁᓵᔅ ᒉᒌ ᐃᔥᐱᔥ ᓯᒋᑦ ᐊᐧᐁᓐ, ᐁᒄᔥ ᐁᑳ
ᒉᒋᒻ ᒋᐳᐱᑕᐦᒃ ᓂᐸᐃᐲᔑᒻ ᒌ ᐃᑌᔨᐦᑕᒻ᙮
ᐅᒎᓐ ᒫᒃ ᑲᔦ᙮ ᒥᒍᓐ ᒋᐱᐦᒌ ᒪᓯᓇᐦᐊᒻ ᒉᐧᑳᔫ
ᐊᓂᑕ ᑳ ᐃᔥᐱᔥ ᒌ ᐹᔥᑌᔨᒡ ᐅᑌᔨᓅ᙮ ᐁᒄ
ᑳ ᐃᑎᔨᑦ, ᑲᓇᐧᐋᐸᐦᑕᐦ ᒫ᙮ ᑳ ᐅᐦᒋ ᒋᔅᒋᔨᑦ
ᒥᐦᒉᐧᑖᐤ ᐁᒌ ᓂᑑᐦᐅᑦ ᑳ ᐃᔥᐱᔥ ᐯᒋ

Jonathan descendit du camion, s'approcha d'un buisson, défit son jean et urina dans la neige d'octobre. Il referma son zipper, remonta dans le camion et son père passa la vitesse pour le remettre en marche. Ils roulèrent lentement, cherchant attentivement des traces ou des feuillages dérangés, tout indice qu'un porc-épic ou une perdrix étaient passés par là. Un orignal serait bien. Jonathan n'avait toujours pas abattu un orignal. Il dévissa le bouchon de sa bouteille d'eau et en aspira une gorgée pour se remplir la bouche. Étrange comme sa bouche était sèche. La chasse du matin, une paire d'oies, était posée à l'arrière du camion. Ils repartirent de l'avant.

Sauf que Jonathan avait besoin d'uriner. À nouveau. Son père arrêta le camion.

C'était ridicule.

Il avait uriné *huit* fois au courant de la dernière heure. Comment un corps humain pouvait-il même produire autant d'urine ? Quel était l'intérêt de refermer sa braguette s'il allait à nouveau devoir uriner ? Et sa bouche. Il aurait pu écrire une lettre sur sa langue tant elle était sèche. Concentre-toi, se disait-il. Jonathan avait beaucoup chassé. Il avait abattu sa

Jonathan stepped out of the truck, sidled up to a bush, unzipped his jeans, and peed into the October snow. He zipped up, climbed back into the truck, and his dad slid it into gear again. They drove slowly, looking out carefully for tracks or disturbed foliage, any hint that a porcupine or partridge had passed by. Moose would be nice. Jonathan still hadn't shot a moose. He twisted the cap off his water bottle and sucked back a mouthful. Strange how dry his mouth was. This morning's kill, a pair of geese, sat in the back of the truck. They inched forward again.

Except – Jonathan had to pee. Again. His dad stopped the truck.

This was ridiculous.

He'd peed *eight* times in the last hour. How could one human body even make that much pee? What was the point in doing up his fly if he was just gonna have to pee again? And his mouth. He could write a letter on his tongue, it was so dry. Focus, he told himself. Jonathan had done quite a bit of hunting. Shot his first partridge when he was six. Now, he knew,

ᐧᒑᓂᑲᓐ᙮ ᒨᔥ ᒌᐦ ᓂᑐᐦᐆ ᐧᒑᓂᑲᓐ᙮ ᑯᐧᑖᔥᒡ ᒌᐦ ᐃᐦᑎᐦᑐᐳᐧᓈᓯᐤ ᓃᔥᑎᒻ ᑳ ᓂᐱᐦᐋᑦ ᐱᔮᐤᐦ᙮ ᐅᔮ ᒫᒃ ᐊᓅᐦᒡ, ᒌᐦ ᒋᔅᒑᔨᐦᑎᒻ ᓈᔥᒡ ᒑ ᓈᓂᑎᐧᐋᐱᑦ = ᒥᒄ ᒫᒃ ᓈᔥᒡ ᐋᑳ ᐅᐦᒋ ᒥᔪᒥᒋᐦᐅᑦ᙮

ᐋᐦ ᐹᔥᑖᔨᒡ ᐊᐧᐋᓐ ᐅᑐᓐ᙮ ᐋᓯᐦᒡ ᐋᐦ ᓯᒋᑦ᙮ ᒌᐦ ᐧᐋᐱᑎᒻ ᐋᐦ ᒥᓯᓈᑖᔨᐤ ᐅᔮ ᐧᐄᔮᔥᑖᐦ᙮ ᐅᐧᐋ, ᐊᓂᑎᐦ ᐋᐦ ᒥᔖᔨᒡ ᒥᓯᓂᐦᐄᑭᓈᒋᓂᔨᐤ = ᐋᐦ ᔖᑳᐅᐱᔨᓈᓂᐧᐃᐧᐃᔨᒡ ᐋᐦ ᐋᔨᒨᑖᔨᒡ᙮ ᒌᐦ ᐊᐧᐋᔑᔒᐤ ᐧᒑᓂᑲᓐ ᑭᔮᐦ ᒌᐦ ᒥᔫᔮᔭᐦᒌ ᑭᔮᐦ ᒌᐦ ᒥᔪᐱᒫᑎᓰᐤ᙮ ᒌᐦ ᓂᔮᔪᔖᐳᐳᐧᓈᓯᐤ, ᒌᐦ ᓂᑐᐦᐆ ᑭᔮᐦ ᒌᐦ ᒋᔅᑯᑎᒫᓰ ᑳ ᐄᔥᐹᔨᒡ ᒋᔅᑯᑎᒫᑑᑭᒥᑯᐦᒡ ᑭᔮᐦ ᒌᐦ ᐧᐄᒋᐦᐋᐤ ᑭᔮᐦ ᒌᐦ ᓈᑎᒧᐧᐋᐤ ᒥᔅᑎᓯᓃ ᐯᕽᔅ ᐋᐦ ᐧᐋᐧᐋᐹᔅᑯᐦᐄᒫᓂᐧᐃᐧᐃᔨᒡ᙮ ᓂᒧᐃ ᔖᑳᐅᐱᔨᒥᒑ᙮

ᒋᑭ ᒌᐦ ᐄᔑᓈᑯᓂᔨᐧᐋ ᒫᒃ ᐅᔮ᙮

ᒑᒃ ᐊᓂᑖᐦ ᐹᑎᒫᐦ, ᑳ ᐋᐱᑦ ᐊᓂᑖᐦ ᑭᐦᒋᓂᐦᒡ ᒦᒋᓰᓈᐦᑎᑯᐦᒡ ᐧᒑᓂᑲᓐ ᐋᐦ ᐋᔨᒥᐦᑖᑦ ᐊᓂᑖᐦ ᐋᐦ ᐃᐦᑐᑎᑭᓂᐧᐃᐧᐃᔨᒡ ᐋᐦ ᓂᑑᑎᐹᔨᒦᓯᓈᓂᐧᐃᐧᐃᔨᒡ ᒑ ᔖᑳᐅᐱᔨᐧᑳ ᐊᐧᐋᓐ᙮ ᐊᓂᑖᐦ ᑳ ᐄᔑ ᐲᐦᑖᐦᒃ ᐊᓂᑎᐦ ᒑ ᐱᐦᒋᑭᐧᐃᓂᐦᒃ ᐅᒥᐦᒄ, ᑳ ᑯᐃᑯᓂᐦᒃ ᐊᓂᔮ ᒑ ᒌᔥᑎᐦᐅᓯᐧᐋᒐᑦ ᑭᔮᐦ ᑳ ᒌᔥᑖᐦᒃ ᐹᔨᒃ ᐅᑎᐦᒌ᙮ ᑎᔮᐦᒋᐦᑖᑦ ᐊᐱᔒᔥ ᐅᒥᐦᒃ ᐊᓂᑎᐦ ᐊᓂᔮ ᑳ ᐄᔑ ᐲᐦᑎᐦᐋᔑᑦ ᒑ ᓂᑑᑎᐹᔨᐦᑎᒃ ᐊᓂᔮᐦ ᐋᔥᐱᔑ ᐃᐦᑎᑯᓂᔨᒡ ᔖᑳᔨᐤ ᐅᒥᐦᑯᐦᒡ᙮ ᐊᓂᔮ ᒫᒃ ᑯᐧᑖᔥᒡ ᑭᔮᐦ ᐊᓂᑖᐦ ᐄᔑ ᓃᐦᑖᐦᒡ ᐋᐦ ᐄᔅᐱᔨᔨᒡ ᐋᔪᐧᐃᒄ ᒫᔮᐤ ᐋᔑ ᐃᐦᑎᑯᓂᔨᒡ ᔖᑳᔮᔨᐤ ᐊᐧᐋᓐ ᐅᒥᐦᑯᐦᒡ, ᒌᐦ ᒋᔅᒑᔨᐦᑎᒻ

ᐊᐧᐋᔒᐅᑦ᙮ ᑳ ᑯᐧᑖᓰᐳᓀᓯᑦ ᐁᑯᑦ ᐅᔅᑲᒡ ᑳ ᓂᐸᐦᐋᑦ ᐱᓭᐤ᙮ ᐁᒄ ᒫᒃ ᐊᓅᐦᒌᔥ ᐊᓂᔫ ᒣᐧᑳᒡ ᐁ ᓂᑑᐦᐅᐧᑖᐤ ᐅᐦᑖᐧᐄᐦ ᐁᐅᒄ ᐊᓂᔫ ᒥᒄ ᒋᐹ ᒫᒥᑐᓀᔨᐦᑕᒥᐦᐄᑰ = ᒥᒄ ᒫᒃ ᓇᒧᐃ ᒥᒍᓐ ᐅᐦᒋ ᒥᔫᒪᐦᒋᐦᐆ᙮

ᐁ ᐹᐦᑯᑯᓀᐧᐁᐸᔨᑦ᙮ ᐁ ᐋᐃᐦᑲᒥᓵᑦ᙮ ᓵᔅ ᐊᓂᑌ ᒌ ᐧᐋᐸᐦᑕᒻ ᐅᔫ ᐁ ᐋᔨᒨᑌᔨᒡ ᐧᐃᓭᔅ᙮ ᓇᒧᐃ ᐋ ᐁ ᒪᔑᑲᓂᔨᒡ ᒪᓯᓇᐦᐁᒋᐧᓈᓂᐦᒡ ᐁ ᐋᔨᒨᑌᔨᒡ ᐁ ᔩᐧᐋᑲᒥᐦᐧᑳᓄᔨᒡ᙮ ᒌ ᐊᐧᐋᔑᔫ ᐧᐄ, ᒌ ᒥᔫᔅᑲᐧᐃᔫ ᑲᓭ ᒌ ᒥᔫᑲᓇᐧᐁᔨᒥᔩ᙮ ᒌ ᓂᔮᐃᓄᔖᐳᓀᔩ ᐁᔅᒄ ᑲᓭ ᒌ ᐃᔅᑰᓅ ᑲᓭ ᒌ ᒣᑐᐧᐁᐤ ᒪᔅᑯᒦᐦᒡ ᐁ ᐸᐹᒥᔅᑯᐸᔨᓈᓄᔨᒡ᙮ ᓇᒧᐃ ᓈᓂᑑ ᓂᔩᐧᐋᑲᒥᐦᐧᑫᓈᒣ ᓃᔮ ᐧᐄ, ᒌ ᐃᑌᔨᐦᑕᒻ᙮

ᓇᒧᐃ ᑳᑲᓭ ᑖᐧᐯ ᓂᔩᐧᐋᑲᒥᐦᐧᑫ, ᒌ ᐃᑌᔨᐦᑕᒻ ᒣᒃ᙮

ᓇᒧᐃ ᒥᐦᒣᑐ ᒌᔑᑳᐤ ᐊᓂᑕ ᐊᓂᔫ ᑳ ᓂᑑᐦᐅᐧᑖᐤ ᐅᐦᑖᐧᐄ, ᒦᒋᓰᓈᐦᑎᑯᐦᒡ ᐁ ᐊᐱᑦ ᒌ ᐊᔨᒥᐦᑖᐤ ᒪᓯᓇᐦᐄᑲᓂᔫ ᐁ ᐧᐄᐦᑕᒧᐧᐋᑲᓅᑦ ᑖᓐ ᒣ ᐃᐦᑑᑕᐦᒃ ᐊᓂᔫ ᒣ ᐋᐸᒋᐦᑖᑦ ᒣᒌ ᐅᐦᒋ ᒋᔅᒣᔨᐦᑖᑯᓂᔨᒡ ᐁ ᔩᐧᐋᑲᒥᐦᐧᑫᐧᑫ᙮ ᑳ ᐅᑎᓇᐦᒃ ᐊᓂᔫ ᑳ ᒌᑕᐧᐁᑲᔑᔨᒡ ᑳ ᒥᔅᑕᐱᔖᔑᔨᒡ ᒪᓯᓇᐦᐁᒋᐧᓈᓂᔑᔫ ᐁᒄ ᑳ ᒉᑯᐦᐊᐦᒃ ᐊᓂᑕ ᐊᓂᔫ ᒋᐹ ᒉᑯᐦᑕᑖᔖ, ᐁᒄ ᑲᓭ ᑳ ᐸᒋᔥᑲᐦᐊᔑᑦ ᐯᔭᒄ ᐅᑎᐦᒌ ᐁ ᐋᐸᒋᐦᑖᑦ ᐊᓂᔫ ᐸᒋᔥᑲᐦᐅᐧᐋᑲᓂᔫ᙮ ᑳ ᐊᔕᐦᐊᔑᑦ ᐊᓂᔫ ᐅᒥᐦᒄ ᐊᓂᑕ ᐊᓂᔫ ᑳ ᒥᔅᑲᐧᐁᑲᔑᔨᒡ ᒪᓯᓇᐦᐁᒋᐧᓈᓂᔑᔫ᙮ ᓃᐦᑖᐦᒡ 6 ᐁ ᐃᐦᑕᑯᓂᔨᒡ ᐊᐧᐁᓐ ᐅᔖᑲᒻ ᒧᔮᒻ ᐃᔑᓈᑯᓂᔫ, ᒋᔅᑑᒡ 6 ᒫᒃ

première perdrix à six ans. Il savait que c'était le moment de se concentrer, mais il se sentait *affreusement mal*.

was the time to concentrate – but he felt *awful*.

La bouche sèche. Miction fréquente. Il avait vu ces mots quelque part sur une liste. Non, sur un poster à propos... du diabète ? Jonathan était jeune, en forme et en bonne santé. Un chasseur de 15 ans, lycéen et homme fort de l'équipe de hockey des Bears de Mistissini. Ça ne pouvait pas être le diabète.

Dry mouth. Frequent urination. He'd seen those words somewhere on a list. No, on a poster about – diabetes? Jonathan was young and fit and healthy. A 15-year-old hunter and high school student and enforcer on the Mistissini Bears hockey team. It couldn't be diabetes.

Si ?

Could it?

Quelques jours plus tard, Jonathan s'assit à la table de la cuisine et lut les instructions sur une trousse de dépistage du diabète. Il inséra une bandelette d'analyse dans le glucomètre, déballa la lancette de la trousse et se piqua le doigt. Il étala soigneusement un peu de sang sur la bandelette de test. Il savait qu'un taux de glycémie inférieur à 6 était normal, qu'entre 6 et 7 se situait le prédiabète (un signe avant-coureur du diabète), et que tout ce qui dépassait 7 était du diabète.

A few days later, Jonathan sat at the kitchen table and read the instructions on a diabetes test kit. He inserted a test strip into the glucometer device, unwrapped the lancet in the kit, and pricked his finger. He carefully smeared some blood onto the test strip. A blood sugar level below 6 was normal, he knew, between 6 and 7 was pre-diabetes, a warning sign that diabetes was just around the corner, and anything over 7 was diabetes.

ᐅᔮ, ᐊᓂᔮ ᒫᒃ ᑯᐧᑖᔥᒡ ᑭᔮᐦ ᓃᐧᓲᔥᒡ ᐋᐦ ᐄᐦᑎᑯᓂᔨᒡ ᐋᔪᐧᐃᒄ ᒑᑳᑦ ᓲᔥ ᐋᐦ ᓲᑳᐅᐱᔨᑦ ᐊᐧᐋᓐ, ᐋᐦ ᐧᐄᐦᑎᒫᑯᑦ ᒑ ᓈᓈᑭᒋᐦᐄᓯᑦ ᐋᑳ ᒑ ᒌᐦ ᓲᑳᐅᐱᔨᑦ ᐊᓂᑖᐦ ᐄᔑ ᓃᔥᑖᒥᐦᒡ, ᑭᔮᐦ ᒫᒃ ᐄᔥᐱᒥᐦᒡ ᓃᐧᓲᔥᒡ ᐋᐦ ᐄᐦᑎᑯᓂᐅᒡ ᐋᔪᐧᐃᒄ ᓲᔥ ᐋᔮᑦ ᑳᓲᑳᐱᔨᓈᓂᐧᐃᐧᐃᔨᒡ᙮

ᑳᓂᐧᐋᐱᐦᑎᐦᒃ ᐊᓂᔮ ᒑ ᐧᐄᐦᑎᒫᑯᑦ ᐋᔥᐱᔥ ᐃᐦᑎᑯᓂᔨᒡ ᓲᑳᔨᐤ ᐅᒥᐦᑯᐦᒡ᙮ ᐊᐧᑳᒋᔥᑖᔨᒡ 32᙮2᙮ ᓂᒧᐃ ᓈᓂᑎᐤ ᑖᐧᐹᒥᑭᔨᒋᒑ᙮ ᐊᓂᔮ ᐊᐅᔥᑖᐦ ᓂᔥᑐᒥᑎᓂᐤ ᐋᐦ ᐄᔅᐱᔨᔨᒡ ᐊᐧᐋᓐ ᒋᑭ ᒌᐦ ᓂᐹᐤ ᑭᔮᐦ ᓂᒥ ᒋᑭ ᒌᐦ ᑯᔥᑯᓈᑭᓂᐆ ᑭᔮᐦ ᑏᐧᐋᐦᒡ ᐲᐦᑎᑭᐦᐋᑭᓂᐆ ᓂᑐᐦᑯᔨᓂᑭᒥᑯᐦᒡ᙮ ᒦᓐ ᓈᑑᑎᐹᔨᐦᑎᐦᒃ ᐋᔪᐧᐃᒄ 32᙮1 ᐊᔅᐱᔨᔨᒡ᙮ ᒥᓐ ᓂᔥᑖᐤ ᓈᑑᒋᔅᒑᔨᑎᐦᒃ ᐅᒥᐦᒄ᙮ ᐋᔑᒄ ᐃᔮᐱᒡ ᐊᐧᑳᔅᐱᔨᔨᒡ᙮ ᓂᒧᐃ ᒋᑭ ᒌᐦ ᐋᐧᓈᐦᑎᒼ ᐧᒑᓂᑲᓐᒼ ᑭᔨᐧᐹ ᑖᐧᐹᐦ ᐋᔮᑦ ᐋᐦ ᓲᑳᐅᐱᔨᓈᐃᐧᐃᐧᐃᔨᒡ᙮

ᓈᐳᐧᐃᑦ, ᓂᑐᐦᑯᔨᓂᑭᒥᑯᐦᒡ ᐋᑐᐦᑖᑦ, ᑏᐧᐋᐦᒡ ᒌᐦ ᒌᔥᑎᐦᐧᐋᑭᓂᐆ ᐃᓐᓯᓕᓐ᙮ ᐹᔨᐧᑳᐤ ᐋᐦ ᒌᓂᐧᑳᓂᐦᑖᔨᒡᐦ ᐲᓯᒨᑳᓐᐦ ᑳ ᐄᔥᐱᔑ ᒌᔥᑎᐦᐧᐋᑭᓂᐧᐃᑦ ᐄᓐᓯᓕᓐ ᓲᔥ ᓈᔥᒡ ᐄᔨᐦᒡ ᐄᑎᒥᒋᐦᐆ.

ᐊᓅᐦᒡ ᒫᒃ ᒫᐧᑳᒡ ᐅᔥᑖᐱᔨᐤ: ᐊᓂᔮ ᐋᔅᐱᔨᔨᒡ ᐋᐦ ᓲᑳᐅᐱᔨᑦ ᐋᔪᐧᐃᒄ ᐋᔑ ᐧᐄᐦᑎᒫᒑᐱᔨᔨᒡ ᐊᓂᑖᐦ ᔑᐳᑯᒨ ᓂᑐᐦᑯᔨᓂᑭᒥᑯᐦᒡ ᒑ ᐃᐦᑖᑯᐱᓈ ᐊᓂᑎᐦ ᒑ ᓈᓈᑭᒋᐦᐄᑯᑦ ᓂᑐᐦᑯᔨᓐᐦ ᑭᔮᐦ ᓂᑐᐦᑯᔨᓂᔅᐧᑳᐤᐦ᙮ ᐊᓂᑖᐦ ᓂᑐᐦᑯᔨᓈᐱᑎᓰᐧᐃᓂᐦᒡ ᐋᑯᑖᐦ ᐋᔑ ᐋᐱᑎᓯᔨᒡᐦ ᐅᑳᐧᐄᐦ, ᒌᐦ ᒋᔅᒑᔨᐦᑎᒼ ᔮᔨᑖ ᒑ

7 ᐁ ᐃᐦᑕᑯᓂᔨᒡ ᐁᑯᑦ ᐧᐁᐦᒋ ᒋᔅᑫᔨᐦᑖᑯᓂᔨᒡ ᑫᒌ ᓰᐧᐋᑲᓂᐦᐧᑫᑦ, ᐁᒄ ᐅᔥᑌ 7 ᐃᐦᑕᑯᓂᔨᑫ ᓵᔅ ᒋᐦᒋᐧᐁ ᓰᐧᐋᑲᒥᐦᐧᑫᐤ᙮

ᑳ ᑲᓇᐧᐋᐸᐦᑕᐦᒃ ᐊᓂᑌ ᒣᓯᓈᑌᔨᒡ ᑖᓂᑕ ᐁ ᐃᐦᑕᑯᓂᔨᒡ ᐅᒥᐦᒄ᙮ 32.2 ᒌ ᐃᒋᔥᑌᔫ᙮ ᓇᒧᐃ ᐅᐦᒋ ᐧᐄ ᑖᐯᐦᑕᒼ᙮ ᐅᔥᑌ 30 ᐁ ᐃᔅᐱᔥ ᓲᑳᐅᐸᔨᒡ ᐅᒥᐦᒄ ᑏᐧᐁᐦᒡ ᐋᐦᑯᓰᐅᑲᒥᑯᐦᒡ ᒋᐹ ᐃᑎᔑᐦᐧᐋᑲᓅ ᐧᐁᔅ ᒋᑲᒌ ᐃᔑᓈᑯᓂᔫ ᑫᒌ ᐋᑯᐧᐁᔨᐦᑕᐦᒃ ᐁᑳ ᑏᐧᐁᐦᒡ ᑫᒌ ᐋᐱᔥᑯᔑᑦ᙮ ᒦᓐ ᑳ ᐃᐦᑑᑕᐦᒃ ᐊᓂ᙮ 32.1᙮ ᒦᓐ ᑳ ᐃᐦᑑᑕᐦᒃ, ᑫᒃ ᒥᐦᑫᐧᑖᐤ ᑳᐦ ᐃᐦᑑᑕᐦᒃ ᐁᑯᓐ ᔮᐸᒡ ᑳ ᐃᒋᔥᑌᔨᒡ᙮ ᑖᐧᐯ ᑮᐹ, ᒌ ᓰᐧᐋᑲᒥᐦᐧᑫ ᑖᐧᐯ᙮

ᒌ ᐸᔑᑰ ᐊᓂᑕ ᑳ ᐊᐱᑦ ᐁᒄ ᓂᑐᐦᑯᐃᓂᑲᒥᑯᐦᒡ ᑳ ᐃᑐᐦᑌᑦ, ᑳ ᐸᒋᔥᑲᐦᐧᐋᑲᓅᑦ ᐊᓂᔫ ᑳᒌ ᐸᒋᔥᑲᐦᐧᐋᑲᓅᑦ ᐊᐧᐁᓐ ᐁ ᓰᐧᐋᑲᒥᐦᐧᑫᑦ, ᐃᓐᓯᓕᓐ ᑳ ᐃᔑᓂᐦᑳᑌᒡ᙮ ᐯᔭᐧᑳᐤ ᑳᐦ ᒌᓂᐧᑳᓂᐦᑌᔨᒡ ᐧᐋᒡ ᓵᔅ ᐊᐱᓃ ᒌ ᐃᑕᒪᐦᒋᐦᐆ᙮

ᒌ ᐃᐦᑕᑯᓂᔫ ᒫᒃ ᑫᐧᑳᔫ ᑖᓐ ᑳ ᐃᔑ ᐅᔥᑕᐧᐁᔨᐦᑕᒥᐦᐄᑯᑦ: ᒌ ᒋᔅᑫᔨᐦᑕᒼ ᐊᓂᔫ ᐁ ᐃᔥᐱᔥ ᓲᑳᐅᐸᔨᑦ ᑫᔥᑎᓈᔥ ᔑᐴᑲᒨ ᐋᐦᑯᓰᐅᑲᒥᑯᐦᒡ ᒋᑲ ᑲᓇᐧᐁᔨᒫᑲᓅ ᐊᓂᑌ ᑫ ᓇᓈᑲᒋᐦᐄᑯᑦ ᓂᑐᐦᑰᐃᓐ ᑲᔦ ᓂᑐᐦᑰᐃᓂᔅᐧᑫᐤᐦ᙮ ᓂᑐᐦᑯᐃᓂᑲᒥᑯᐦᒡ ᒌ ᐋᐸᑎᓯᔫᐦ ᐅᑳᐧᐄᐦ ᒌ ᑫᔅᑎᓈᐦᐆ ᑫ ᐋᔨᐦᑲᒥᐦᐄᑯᑦ ᐋᐦᑯᓰᐅᑲᒥᑯᐦᒡ

Il regarda le glucomètre. Il indiquait que son taux de sucre dans le sang était de 32,2. Cela ne *pouvait* être possible. Un résultat de plus de 30 signifiait qu'il devait être hospitalisé immédiatement parce qu'il pourrait tomber dans le coma. Il refit le test. 32.1. Il le refit encore et encore, et encore. Tous les chiffres étaient à peu près les mêmes. Aucun doute, Jonathan était diabétique.

He looked at the glucometer. It said his blood sugar level was 32.2. That *couldn't* be right. A reading of over 30 meant he had to be hospitalized immediately because he could slip into a coma. He took the test again. 32.1. And again and again and again. All the numbers were about the same. No question, Jonathan had diabetes.

Il se leva de sa chaise et se rendit à la clinique, où on lui injecta de l'insuline. Une heure plus tard, il se sentait mieux.

He got up from his chair, went to the clinic, where they injected him with insulin. An hour later, he felt better.

Toutefois, il avait désormais un problème : son taux de glycémie signifiait qu'il devrait être à l'hôpital de Chibougamau où les médecins et les infirmières pourraient le mettre en observation. Sa mère était une représentante en santé communautaire (RSC), et elle l'obligerait

But now he had a problem: his blood sugar levels meant that he should be in the Chibougamau hospital where the doctors and nurses could watch him. His mother was a Community Health Representative (CHR), and she would make him go, he was sure – and that

ᓂᐦᐋᔨᐦᑎᐦᒃ ᐊᓂᑖᐦ ᒑ ᐃᐦᑖᑯᐱᓈ = ᑭᔮᐦ ᒌᐦ ᒋᔅᒑᔨᐦᑎᒻ ᒑ ᐧᐃᔥᑖᐲᐦᐄᑯᑦ ᐋᑳ ᒑ ᒌᐦ ᐄᔅᐱᔨᑦ ᐊᓂᔮ ᒑ ᐄᔥᐧᑳᑎᐧᐃᔥᑖᔨᒡ ᐊᓂᑖᐦ ᑳ ᐧᐄᐦ ᐄᔅᐱᔨᑦ᙮ ᒌᐦ ᐧᐄᐦ ᐧᐄᒑᐧᐋᐤ ᐊᓂᔮᐦ ᐅᐧᐄᒑᐧᐋᑭᓐᐦ ᐊᓂᔮᐦ ᑳ ᒫᑎᐧᐋᒫᑦ ᐋᐦ ᑑᐦᐧᐋᑦ ᐊᓂᑖᐦ ᒌᐦ ᐧᐄᐦ ᐄᔅᐱᔨᔪᐧᐃᒡ ᐧᒫᓐᑎᓈᐧᔮᑦ ᒑ ᓂᑑᓈᓈᑭᒋᐦᐄᐧᐋᒡ ᐋᐦ ᒫᑎᐧᐋᓂᐧᐃᔨᒡ, ᐊᓂᔮᐦ ᐧᒫᓐᑎᓈᐧᔮᑦ ᐋᒍᐧᐁᑦᔅ ᐋᐦ ᒫᑎᐧᐋᔨᒡᐦ ᑭᔮᐦ ᒑ ᓂᑑᓂᒋᔥᑭᐧᐋᒡ ᒌᔑᒫᐧᐋᔨᒋᐦᐋ᙮ ᐊᓂᔮᐦ ᒫᒃ ᑳ ᐧᐋᐱᓈᔨᒡᐦ ᑑᐦᐋᓐᐦ ᐋᔪᐧᐃᑯᓐᐦ ᒋᐱᐦ ᐧᐄᒋᒦᒋᓯᒪᐤ ᐧᒑᓂᔕᓐ ᑭᔮᐦ ᒋᐱᐦ ᐅᔑᐦᑖᑭᓂᐧᐃᐧᐃᔨᐤ ᑖᐱᔥᑯᓐ ᒑ ᓅᑯᓯᒡ ᐋᐦ ᑎᑳᔥᑖᐱᔨᔨᒡ᙮ ᒋᔥᒋᐧᐋ ᒌᐦ ᐄᑖᔨᐦᑖᑯᓂᔨᐤ ᐅᔮ ᑭᔮᐦ ᔮᔨᑖ ᒌᐦ ᐧᐄᐦ ᐃᐦᑐᑎᒻ᙮

ᓈᔥᒡ ᒥᒋᓐ ᐋᐦ ᐧᐄᐦᑎᒧᐧᐋᑦ, ᑭᔮᐦ ᐋᐦ ᓂᑎᐧᐋᔨᒫᑦ ᔮᔨᑖ ᒑ ᐃᔮᐱᓯᐦᑖᑯᑦ ᐅᑳᐧᐄᐦ, ᓈᔥᒡ ᓲᐦᒃ ᐋᐦ ᑯᒋᔥᑖᑦ ᒑ ᓂᐦᐋᔨᒥᑯᑦ ᒑ ᒌᐦ ᒋᔥᒋᐱᔨᑦ᙮ ᔮᔨᑖ ᒑ ᑎᐦᑯᓂᐦᒃ ᔖᐳᓂᑭᓐᐦ ᑭᔮᐦ ᐃᓐᓯᓴᓐ, ᐄᑖᐤ ᐊᓂᔮᐦ ᐅᑳᐧᐄᐦ᙮ ᓈᔥᒡ ᒑ ᓈᓈᑭᒋᐦᑖᑦ ᐊᓂᔮ ᒑ ᐄᔑ ᒌᔥᑎᐦᐅᓯᑯᐱᓈ᙮ ᒥᐦᒑᑖᐤ ᒑ ᒥᓯᓂᐦᐋᒧᐧᐋᑦ ᑳ ᐱᐹᑎᐦᑯᓂᑭᓂᐧᐃᔑᔨᒡ ᐋᐦ ᐋᐱᒋᐦᑖᑦ ᑭᔮᐦ ᒑ ᐧᐄᐦᑎᒧᐧᐋᑦ ᐋᑎ ᐃᔨᐦᑎᒃ ᐊᓂᔮ ᒑ ᐊᑎ ᐄᔥᐧᑳᑎᐧᐃᔥᑖᔨᒡ᙮ ᑭᔮᐦ ᑳᐦ ᐄᑖᑦ ᐋᑳ ᒑ ᐃᔮᔨᒫᔨᐦᑎᒥᐦᐋᑦ, ᑭᔮᐦ ᑯᐃᔅᒄ ᒑ ᑭᓂᐧᐋᔨᒦᓯᑦ᙮ ᐋᑦ ᒫᒃ ᐄᔅᐱᔨᐦᐄᑯᒐ ᒐᐧᑳᔨᐤ, ᐃᐦᑎᑯᓐ ᓂᑐᐦᑯᔨᓂᑭᒥᒄᐦ ᐊᓂᑖᐦ ᐧᒫᓐᑎᓈᐧᔮᑦ᙮ ᒑᒃ ᒫᒃ ᐄᔨᐧᐋ ᑳ ᐃᔮᐱᓯᐦᑖᑯᑦ ᒑ ᒌᐦ ᐧᐄᒋᐦᐄᐧᐋᑦ ᐊᓂᔮᐦ ᐅᑳᐧᐄᐦ᙮

ᒥᒄ ᒫᒃ ᐋᔥᒄ ᒌᐦ ᐃᐦᑎᑯᓂᔨᐤ ᒐᐧᑳᔨᐤ ᐋᑳ ᒥᔪᐱᔨᐦᐄᑯᑦ, ᐋᔪᐧᐃᒄ: ᓂᒧᐃ ᐅᐦᒋ

ᒉᒌ ᐃᐦᑖᑦ ᐁᒄ ᑮᐹ ᓇᒧᐃ ᒋᐹᐦᒌ ᐃᐦᑑ ᐊᓂᔫ ᑳᐧᐄ ᐃᐦᑎᑦ ᐊᓂᔫ ᒉ ᐃᔅᐧᑳᐤ ᑑᔥᑌᔨᒡ᙮ ᐅᐧᐄᒉᐧᐋᑲᓐ ᑳ ᐧᐄᒋᒣᑐᐧᐁᒫᑦ ᑑᐦᐋᓐ ᑳ ᑕᐦᒋᔥᑯᐧᐋᑲᓅᔨᒡ ᐁᐃᔑ ᒣᑐᐧᐁᐧᑖᐤ ᒨᓴᔮᐦᒡ ᒌᐧᐄ ᐃᔅᐸᔫᒡ ᒉᒌ ᓂᑑ ᑲᓇᐧᐋᐸᒫᐧᑖᐤ ᒪᑎᓇᔨᑦ ᐋᒍᐧᐁᑦᔅ ᐁ ᒥᑐᐧᐁᔨᐦᑖᐤ ᐁᒄ ᑲᔦ ᒥᓯᐧᐁ ᒌᐧᐄ ᓇᒋᔅᑲᐧᐁᐅᒡ ᐊᓂᔫᐦ ᒣᑐᐧᐁᓲᐦ᙮ ᒋᐹ ᐧᐄᒋᒦᒋᓲᒣᐤ ᐊᓂᔫ ᐯᔭᒄ ᑳ ᓃᑳᓀᔨᐦᑖᑯᓯᔨᒡ ᒣᑐᐧᐁᓲ ᑲᔦ ᒋᐹ ᒪᓯᓈᐅᐸᔨᐦᐋᑲᓅᐧᐃᒡ ᐁ ᓃᔑᐧᑖᐤ᙮ ᒋᐦᒋᐧᐁ ᒌ ᐃᑌᔨᐦᑕᒥᐦᐄᑰ ᓇᒧᐃ ᒫᒃ ᐅᐦᒋ ᐧᐄ ᐸᑕᐦᐊᒻ ᐅᔫ ᑳᐧᐄ ᐃᐦᑎᐧᑖᐤ᙮

ᑳ ᐊᔨᒥᐦᐋᑦ ᐅᑳᐧᐄ ᐁᐧᐄ ᔖᑯᒋᒫᑦ ᒉᒌ ᐸᒋᔥᑎᓂᑯᑦ ᒨᓴᔮᐦᒡ ᒉᒌ ᐃᔅᐸᔨᑦ᙮ ᒋᐹ ᐊᔮᐤ ᐅᐸᒋᔥᑲᐦᐄᑲᓐᐦ ᑲᔦ ᐅᓂᑐᐦᑯᐃᓈᐳᒻ ᒌ ᐃᑌᐤ᙮ ᒋᐹ ᐸᒋᔅᑲᐦᐆᓲ ᑕᐦᐧᑖᐤ ᒋᐹ ᐸᒋᔅᑲᐦᐆᓲ ᒣᔑᑯᒻ ᒌᔑᑳᐤ᙮ ᑲᔦ ᒋᐹ ᒪᓯᓇᐦᐊᒧᐧᐁᐤ ᐅᑖᐦᑲᐱᐦᒉᓂᑲᓐᔥ ᐁ ᐋᐸᒋᐦᑖᑦ ᒉ ᐃᔥᐱᐦᑕᓂᐦᐅᑦ ᒉ ᐧᐄᐦᑕᒧᐧᐋᑦ ᑖᓐ ᐁ ᐃᐦᑎᑦ᙮ ᓇᒧᐃ ᒋᐹ ᐅᐦᒋ ᐧᐄ ᓭᒋᓯᔫ ᐧᐁᔅ ᒋᐹ ᒥᔫᑲᓇᐧᐁᔨᒥᓲ, ᐁᑳ ᐧᐃᔦᔅ ᒉ ᐅᐦᒋ ᐃᔅᐸᔨᑦ᙮ ᐋᑦ ᒉᐧᑳᔫ ᐃᔅᐸᔨᑦ ᒥᓯᐧᐋᒡ ᐃᐦᑕᑯᓐᐦ ᐋᐦᑯᓰᐅᑲᒥᒄᐦ ᒨᓴᔮᐦᒡ, ᒌᔑ ᐊᔨᒥᐦᐁᐤ ᐊᓂᔫ ᐅᑳᐧᐄ᙮ ᑖᐧᐯ ᒫᒃ ᒌ ᔖᑯᒋᒣᐤ᙮

ᒥᒄ ᒫᒃ ᔮᐸᒡ ᒦᓐ ᑯᑕᒋᔫ ᒉᐧᑳᔫ ᒌ ᐅᔥᑖᐸᔨᐦᐄᑰ᙮ ᓇᒧᐃ ᐅᐦᒋ ᓂᑐᐧᐁᔨᐦᑕᒻ

à s'y rendre, il en était sûr – et cela ruinerait ses plans de fin de semaine. Quelques amis de son camp de football et lui devaient aller à Montréal pour voir le match des Alouettes de Montréal et ensuite rencontrer tous les joueurs. Jonathan souperait avec le quart-arrière et filmerait une annonce avec lui. C'était une opportunité importante et il ne voulait pas la manquer.

would ruin his weekend plans. He and some friends from football camp were going to Montréal to watch the Montréal Alouettes game and then all meet with them. Jonathan would have supper with the quarterback and be in a commercial with him. It was a big deal and he didn't want to miss it.

Méthodiquement et avec détermination, il commença à persuader sa mère de le laisser partir pour ce voyage. Il pourrait emporter des seringues et de l'insuline, arguait-il. Il suivrait parfaitement les règles d'injection. Il lui enverrait des messages textes tout au long de la fin de semaine et la tiendrait au courant. Elle n'avait pas à s'inquiéter pour lui, il serait prudent, il irait bien. De plus, si quoi que ce soit devait mal se passer, Montréal avait des hôpitaux. Finalement, elle se laissa convaincre.

Methodically, purposefully, he began to persuade his mom to let him go on the trip. He could take needles and insulin, he reasoned. He would follow the injection rules perfectly. He would text her throughout the weekend and keep her updated. She didn't need to be afraid for him, he'd be careful, he'd be okay. Besides, if anything went wrong, Montréal had hospitals. In the end, she came around.

Il avait cependant un autre problème : il devait garder son diabète secret. Il

He still had another problem, though: he needed to keep the diabetes secret.

ᓂᑎᐧᐋᔨᐦᑎᒻ ᐋᐦ ᔖᑳᐅᐱᔨᑦ ᒑ ᒋᔅᒑᔨᐦᑎᒥᔨᒡᐦ ᐊᐧᐋᔨᐤᐦ᙮ ᓈᔥᒡ ᑯᐃᔅᑯ ᐋᐦ ᑎᒥᐦᒋᓂᐦᒃ ᐊᓂᔮ ᐅᒌᔥᑎᐦᐅᐧᐋᐳᐃ, ᐊᓂᑖᐦ ᐅᑖᓯᐦᒡ ᐋᑯᑖᐦ ᐋᔑ ᐲᐦᑖᐦᒃ ᑭᔮᐦ ᒦᓐ ᐊᓂᑖᐦ ᐅᐲᐦᑑᐲᒌᔅᓂᐦᒡ ᐋᑯᑎᐦ ᐧᐋᔅᐧᑳᔮᒋᓂᐦᒃ, ᓈᑖᐦ ᐄᑖᒥᐦᒡ ᐧᐄᐅᑎᐦᒡ ᐋᔑ ᐲᐦᑖᐦᒃ, ᐊᓂᑎᐦ ᐋᑳ ᒑ ᒌᐦ ᐧᐋᐱᐦᑎᒥᔨᒡᐦ ᐊᐧᐋᔨᐤᐦ᙮ ᐊᓂᔮ ᒫᒃ ᑳ ᐄᔥᐧᑳᑎᐧᐃᔥᑖᔨᒡ ᑳ ᐄᔑᔨᐧᐄᑦ ᐋᐦ ᒥᓯᓂᐦᐋᒧᐧᐋᑦ ᐅᑳᐧᐄᐦ ᐋᐦ ᑯᐧᑳᒋᒫᑦ ᒑᐧᑳᔨᐤ᙮ ᐄᔅᑯᐱᔨᔨᐧᐋ ᐊᐧᐋᓐ ᐅᔖᑳᒼ ᐋᐦ ᒧᐧᐋᑦ ᑐᔅᑦ, ᐲᐦᐧᓵᔮᔨᐦᑯᓈᐤᐦ ᐋᐦ ᐱᐦᑭᓯᔨᒡᐦ᙮ (ᐄᐦᐄ) ᐋᐦ ᒫᒫᑭᒧᔅᒋᐧᐋᓂᐧᐃᒡ ᒫᒃ ᐧᐄ᙮ (ᓂᒥᒫᐦ) ᓂᒧᐃ ᒫᒃ ᐅᐦᒋ ᐧᐄᐦᑎᒧᐧᐋᐤ ᐊᐧᐋᔨᐤᐦ ᐋᐦ ᔖᑳᐅᐱᔨᑦ, ᓂᒧᐃ ᐅᐦᒋ ᐧᐄᐦᑎᒧᐧᐋᐤ ᐅᐧᐄᒑᐧᐋᑭᓈᐦ, ᐊᓂᔮᐦ ᑳ ᐧᐃᔨᐱᔨᐦᑖᔨᒡᐦ ᐋᐦ ᐱᐹᒥᐱᔨᒡ, ᑭᔮᐦ ᒫᔑᐧᐄᐦ ᐊᓂᔮᐦ ᑳ ᐧᐋᐱᓈᔨᒡᐦ ᑑᐦᐋᓐ ᐧᒫᓂᑎᓅᐧᔮᑦ ᐋᑐᐁᑦᔅ ᑳ ᐧᐄᒋᐦᐋᔨᒡᐦ᙮ ᑭᔮᐦ ᓂᒧᐃ ᐅᐦᒋ ᐅᑎᓂᒻ ᐃᓐᓯᓄᓐ ᐊᓂᔮᐦ ᒑ ᐄᔥᐱᔑ ᐅᑎᓂᒧᑯᐱᓈ᙮ ᑖᐹ ᐧᐋᐦᑎᓐ ᐋᐦ ᒌᔥᑎᐦᐅᓯᓈᓂᐧᐃᒡ, ᐃᑏᓰ᙮ ᐊᓂᑖᐦ ᐋᑳ ᐃᐦᑖᔨᒡᐦ ᐅᓵᐲᐅᑖᓐᐦ ᐋᑯᑖᐦ ᐋᔑ ᒌᔥᑎᐦᐅᓯᑦ ᐊᐧᐋᓐ, ᒫᑎᐧᐋᓰ ᐧᐋᔥ ᓃᔨ᙮ ᓈᔥᑖᐧᐹᐦ ᓅᔅᐲᐅᑖᓐ, ᓂᒧᐃ ᓂᑖᐦᒋᐳᓐ᙮ ᒥᒄ ᒫᒃ, ᐋᔭᐧᐃᒄ ᐧᐋᐦᒋ ᐋᑳ ᐅᐦᒋ ᒌᔥᑎᐦᐅᓯᑦ ᐋᑳ ᐅᐦᒋ ᓂᑎᐧᐋᔨᐦᑎᐦᒃ ᒑ ᐧᐋᐱᒥᑯᑦ ᐊᐧᐋᔨᐤᐦ ᐋᐦ ᐋᐱᒋᔥᑖᑦ ᐃᓐᓯᓄᓂᔨᐤ᙮

ᒋᐦ ᒥᔭᐱᔨᔨᐤ ᐊᓂᔮ ᑳ ᓈᓈᑭᒋᐦᐄᐧᐋᑦ ᐋᐦ ᑑᐦᐊᓂᐧᐃᐧᐃᔨᒡ ᑭᔮᐦ ᓂᒧᐃ ᐅᐦᒋ ᐋᐦᑯᓯᐤ ᐧᒑᓂᑲᑎᓐ, ᒥᒄ ᒫᒃ ᑳ ᐹᒋ ᒌᐧᐋᑦ, ᑏᐧᐋᐦᒡ ᐊᓂᑖᐦ ᐅᓂᐹᐅᑭᒥᑯᐦᒡ ᒌᐦ ᐄᔑ ᐲᐦᒋᒑᐤ ᑭᔮᐦ ᑳ ᐋᐸᐦᒃ ᒑ ᓈᓈᑭᒋᔥᑖᑦ ᐋᐦ ᑎᑳᔥᑖᐱᔨᔨᒡ᙮ ᐋᑯᑖᐦ ᐱᔑᔑᒄ ᑳ ᐃᐦᑖᑦ ᒥᐦᒑᑐ ᒌᔑᑳᐤᐦ᙮

ᑫᒌ ᒋᔅᑫᔨᐦᑕᒥᔨᒡ ᐊᐧᐁᔮᐦ ᐁ ᓰᐧᐋᑲᒥᐦᐧᑫᑦ᙮ ᑳ ᐲᐦᑕᐦᐊᐦᒃ ᐊᓂᔮ ᐅᓂᑐᐦᑯᐃᓈᐴᒻ ᐊᓂᑌ ᐧᐄᐧᐊᑎᐦᒡ, ᐅᑖᓯᐦᒡ ᐁ ᒉᑯᐦᐊᐦᒃ ᐁᒄ ᑳ ᑎᐦᑎᐸᓂᐦᑕᑖᑦ ᐊᓂᔮ ᐅᑖᔅ ᐁᒄ ᐅᐲᐦᑑᐸᐃᒌᔖᓂᐦᒡ ᑳ ᐱᔅᐧᑫᔦᒋᓇᐦᒃ ᐊᓂᔮ ᐅᑖᔅ ᓂᑖᒥᐦᒡ ᐊᓂᑕ ᐊᓂᔮ ᐧᐄᐧᐊᑎᐦᒡ ᑳ ᐃᔑ ᐲᐦᑕᐦᒃ ᐁᑳ ᑮᐹ ᑫᒌ ᐧᐋᐸᐦᑕᒥᔨᒡ ᐊᐧᐁᔮᐦ᙮ ᒣᐧᑳᒡ ᒨᓄᔮᐦᒡ ᑳ ᐃᐦᑖᑦ ᒣᓯᑯᒻ ᒌᔑᑳᐤ ᒌ ᐊᔨᒥᐦᐁᐤ ᐅᑳᐧᐄ ᐁ ᑲᐧᑫᒋᒫᑦ ᒣᐧᑳᔮ᙮ ᓂᑲᒌ ᒧᐧᐋᐤ ᐋ ᐲᔕᐧᐁᐋᐃᐦᑯᓈᐤ ᐁ ᐸᐦᑲᓯᑦ, ᒌᔑ ᑲᐧᑫᒋᒣᐤ᙮ ᐁᐦᐁ᙮ ᐱᒎ ᐧᐄ ᐧᐃᔦᔅ ᐋ ᒋᑲ ᐃᔅᐸᔮ ᓂᔖᑳᒼ ᒫᒫᑯᒪᑫ᙮ ᓇᒧᐃ᙮ ᓇᒧᐃ ᐊᐧᐁᔮᐦ ᐅᐦᒋ ᐧᐄᐦᑕᒧᐧᐁᐤ ᐁ ᓰᐧᐋᑲᒥᐦᐧᑫᑦ, ᓇᒧᐃ ᐅᐦᒋ ᐧᐄᐦᑕᒧᐧᐁᐤ ᐅᐧᐄᒉᐧᐋᑲᓐᐦ, ᓇᒧᐃ ᑲᔦ ᐊᓂᔮᐦ ᑳ ᐱᒥᐸᔨᐦᐄᑯᐧᑖᐤ ᐊᓂᑌ ᑳ ᐃᔅᐸᔨᐧᑖᐤ, ᒣᓯᐧᐄ ᐊᓂᔮᐦ ᒣᑐᐧᐁᓰᐦ ᑫᒌ ᐧᐄᐦᑕᒧᐧᐋᑦ᙮ ᑲᔦ ᒫᒃ ᒌ ᐸᐦᑕᐦᐊᒻ ᐋᔥᑰ ᐁ ᐅᑎᓇᐦᒃ ᐊᓂᔮ ᐅᓂᑐᐦᑯᐃᓂᒻ᙮ ᐋᐃᒥᓐ ᑫᒌ ᐸᒋᔅᑲᐦᐆᓰᔮᓐ, ᒌ ᐃᑌᔨᐦᑕᒻ᙮ ᐊᓂᑌ ᓂᑖᒥᐦᒡ ᓂᔮᔑᒡ ᓂᐹ ᐃᔑ ᐸᒋᔅᑲᐦᐆᓰᓐ ᐊᓂᑕ ᐁ ᐱᒥᔮᔭᓐ᙮ ᒥᒄ ᒫᒃ ᐊᓐ ᐊᐧᐁᓐ ᒨᔥ ᑳ ᓴᓵᐧᐃᔨᑦ ᓃ᙮ ᓂᒥᔮᔅᑲᐧᐃᔨᓐ, ᓇᒧᐃ ᓂᑖᐦᒋᐳᓐ᙮ ᐊᓂᔮ ᑳ ᐃᐦᑎᑦ ᐁᑳ ᐅᐦᒋ ᐃᔥᐱᔥ ᐸᒋᔅᑲᐦᐆᓰᑦ ᓇᒧᐃ ᐅᐦᒋ ᓂᑐᐧᐁᔨᐦᑕᒻ ᑫᒌ ᐧᐋᐸᒫᑲᓅᑦ ᐁ ᐋᔮᑦ ᐊᓂᔮ ᓂᑐᐦᑯᐃᓂᔮ ᐃᓐᓭᓄᓐ ᑳ ᐃᔑᓂᐦᑳᑌᔨᒡ᙮

ᒌ ᒥᔦᔨᐦᑕᒻ ᐊᓂᔮ ᑳ ᒋᐦᒋᐸᔨᐧᑖᐤ ᐅᐧᐄᒋ ᒎᐦᐁᔒᒻ ᐁᑳ ᐅᐦᒋ ᐋᐦᑯᓯᑦ ᒥᒄ ᒫᒃ ᐃᔅᑯᑕᒃ ᑳᐤ ᑳ ᐹᐸᔨᐧᑖᐤ ᑏᐧᐁᐦᒡ ᐅᓂᐯᐅᑲᒥᑯᐦᒡ ᒌ ᐲᐦᑫᐤ ᑳ ᐊᑎ ᐋᐸᐦᐊᐦᒃ ᐊᓂᔮ ᑳᒪᓇᐧᐋᔥᑌᐸᔨᔨᒡ᙮ ᐁᑯᑦ ᐱᔑᒄ ᑳ ᐃᐦᑖᑦ ᒥᐦᑫᑐ ᒌᔑᑳᐤᐦ᙮ ᓇᒧᐃ ᐅᐦᒋ ᐃᑐᐦᑌᐤ

emballa l'insuline avec soin, en la mettant d'abord dans un bas, puis en enroulant les bas dans des sous-vêtements, les rangeant tout au fond de son sac, où personne ne les verrait. Tout au long de la fin de semaine, il envoya fidèlement des messages texte à sa mère pour lui demander conseil. Les toasts affectaient-ils le taux de sucre dans le sang ? (Oui) Un chewing-gum affectait-il le taux de sucre dans le sang ? (Non) Toutefois, il ne mentionna son diabète à personne, ni à ses amis, ni aux organisateurs du voyage, et certainement pas au quart-arrière des Alouettes. Il ne prit pas non plus d'insuline aussi souvent qu'il aurait dû le faire. *Elle est difficile à injecter*, se disait-il. *L'insuline doit aller dans la graisse. Je suis un athlète. Beaucoup de muscles, pas beaucoup de graisse*. Mais en vérité, il ne prenait pas assez d'insuline parce qu'il ne voulait pas être vu avec de l'insuline.

He packed the insulin carefully, tucking it first inside a sock and then rolling the socks into underwear, stuffing it all way down in his bag, where no one would see it. All weekend long, he faithfully texted his mom for advice. Did toast affect blood sugar? (Yes) Did chewing gum affect blood sugar? (No) But he told no one about the diabetes, not his friends, not the trip organizers, and certainly not the Alouettes quarterback. And he didn't take the insulin nearly as often as he should have. *It's hard to inject*, he said to himself. *Insulin has to go into fat. I'm an athlete. Lots of muscle, not a lot of fat.* But in truth, he wasn't taking enough insulin because he didn't want to be seen with insulin.

Le voyage de football s'était bien passé et Jonathan n'était pas tombé malade, toutefois quand il rentra à la maison, il se dirigea directement vers la chambre et alluma la télévision. Et il y resta pendant des jours. Il n'alla pas à l'école. Il n'alla

The football trip was fine and Jonathan didn't get sick, but when he came home, he headed straight for the bedroom and flipped on the TV. And stayed there for days. He didn't go to school. He didn't go to his hockey practices. He didn't go to his

ᓂᒥᒌᔨᐧᐋ ᐅᐦᒋ ᒋᔅᑯᑎᒫᓰ. ᓂᒥᒌᔨᐧᐋ ᐅᐦᒋ ᑯᐧᑳᒋᐦᐄᓰ ᐋᐦ ᐧᐋᐧᐋᐹᔅᑯᐦᐄᒑᓂᐧᐃᐧᐃᔨᒡ. ᓂᒥᒌᔨᐧᐋ ᐅᐦᒋ ᒫᑎᐧᐋᐤ ᒑ ᒌᐦ ᐱᐹᒥᔅᑯᐱᔨᑦ. ᓂᒥᒌᔨᐧᐋ ᐅᐦᒋ ᓂᑎᐧᐋᐱᒫᐤ ᐊᓂᔮᐦ ᐊᐧᐋᔨᐤᐦ ᒑ ᐧᐄᒋᐦᐄᑯᑦ ᐅᐦᒋ ᐊᓂᔮ ᐋᐦ ᔔᑳᐅᐱᔨᑦ.

ᐊᓂᔮ ᒫᒃ ᑳ ᒌᔑᐹᔨᑯᑎᐧᐃᔥᑖᔨᒡ, ᓈᔥᒡ ᐋᐦ ᒌᐦ ᒥᔮᑯᓂᔨᒡ ᐅᓂᐹᐅᑭᒥᒄ.

ᑳ ᒌᔑᓃᔓᑎᐧᐃᔥᑖᔨᒡ, ᐊᐧᑳᑎᑯᑦ ᐅᐦᑖᐧᐄᐦ, ᐧᐋᐱᐦᑎᐦ ᒫ, ᐊᓐ ᒥᒄ ᐋᐦ ᑎᑳᔥᑖᐦᑖᔨᓐ ᓂᒥᔮᐅᑎᐦ ᐊᓂᑎᐦ ᒑ ᒌᐦ ᐅᐦᒋ ᐄᒑᐱᔨᒡ ᐋᐦ ᔔᑳᐅᐱᔨᔨᓐ. ᒋᔅᑯᑎᒫᓯᐦ ᓈᑖᐦ. ᐋᔮᐱᒡ ᒋᑭ ᒌᐦ ᐃᐦᑐᑖᓐ ᐊᓐ ᒥᓯᐧᐋ ᒑᐧᑳᓐ ᑳ ᒌ ᐃᐦᑐᑎᒥᓐ, ᒥᒄ ᐊᓐ ᐧᐋᐦ ᐋᐦ ᐃᐦᑎᔨᓐ ᒋᑭ ᒌᐦ ᐃᐦᑎᓐ, ᒥᒄ ᐋᑲ ᐧᐄᐦ ᒌᔑᐦᑖᔨᓈ ᐊᓐ ᑳ ᐄᔥᐹᒡ ᒋᔅᑯᑎᒫᒐᐧᐃᓐ ᐋᑯᑖᐦ ᐅᑖᐦ ᒥᒄ ᐃᔨᐦᑦ. ᓂᒥᔮᐤ ᒑ ᒋᐱᐦᒋᐦᐄᑯᔨᓐ ᐧᐄ ᐊᓐ ᐋᐦ ᔔᑳᐅᐱᔨᔨᓐ ᐊᓂᑎᐦ ᒑ ᒌᐦ ᐅᐦᒋ ᐋᑲ ᐃᐦᑐᑎᒥᓐ ᒥᓯᐧᐋ ᐊᓐ ᒑᐧᑳᓐ ᐊᓂᑖᐦ ᐄᔑ ᐅᑖᐦᒡ ᑳ ᒌ ᐃᐦᑐᑎᒥᓐ."

ᑏᐧᐋᐦᒡ ᐊᓂᔮ ᒦᓐ ᑳᔑᑳᔨᒡ ᒌᐦ ᓂᑑᒋᔅᑯᑎᒫᓰ ᐧᒑᓂᕋᓐ ᑭᔮᐦ ᒦᓐ ᒌᐦ ᒫᑎᐧᐋᐤ ᐋᐦ ᐧᐋᐧᐋᐹᔅᑯᐦᐄᒑᓂᐧᐃᐧᐃᔨᒡ. ᐧᑳᐧᑳᒋᒥᑯᑦ ᐊᓂᔮᐦ ᐅᒋᒫᐤᐦ ᐊᓂᑖᐦ ᒋᔅᑯᑎᒫᑑᑭᒥᑯᐦᒡ ᑖᓐ ᑳ ᐋᔨᐦᑎᒃ. ᐊᐧᑳᑖᑦ, ᓂᑐᐦᑯᔨᓂᑭᒥᑯᐦᒡ ᓂᒌᐦ ᐄᑐᐦᑖᓐ ᑭᔮᐦ ᐋᐅᒄ ᐧᐋᐦᒋ ᐋᑲ ᐅᐦᒋ ᒋᔅᑯᑎᒫᓯᔮᓐ, ᐋᑲ ᓈᔥᑎᔨᒡ ᐧᐄᐦ ᑭᓂᐧᐋᐱᒫᑦ. ᓂᒧᐃ ᐅᐦᒋ ᐧᐄᐦ ᐋᔨᒧᑎᒧᐧᐋᐤ ᐊᓂᔮ ᐧᐄ ᐋᐦ ᔔᑳᐅᐱᔨᑦ.

ᒋᔅᑯᑕᒫᒉᐅᑲᒥᑯᐦᒡ ᒉᒌ ᓂᑑ ᒋᔅᑯᑕᒫᓯᑦ. ᓇᒧᐃ ᐅᐦᒋ ᐃᑐᐦᑌᐤ ᑕᐦᐧᑖᐤ ᒋᐹ ᓯᓰᐧᐃᔫᒡ ᐅᐧᐄᒋ ᒉᑐᐧᐁᓰᒻᐦ ᐦᐧᐋᑮ ᐁ ᒉᑐᐧᐁᐧᑖᐤ. ᓇᒧᐃ ᑲᔦ ᐅᐦᒋ ᐃᑐᐦᑌᐤ ᑕᐦᐧᑖᐤ ᒥᔦᑕᐧᐁᔨᐧᑖᐤ ᒉᒌ ᐧᐄᒋᒉᑐᐧᐁᒫᑦ. ᓇᒧᐃ ᑲᔦ ᐅᐦᒋ ᓂᑐᐧᐋᐸᒉᐤ ᐊᓂᔫ ᓂᑐᐦᑯᐃᓂᔅᐧᑫᐤ ᑳ ᓰᐧᐋᑲᒥᐦᐧᑳᔨᒡ ᐊᐧᐁᔫᐦ ᑳ ᐧᐋᐧᐄᒋᐦᐋᔨᒡ.

ᒉᒃ ᑳ ᒥᔮᐅᐸᔨᔨᒡ ᐯᔭᒄ ᑑᔥᑌᐤᐦ, ᒉᒃ ᓇᒧᐃ ᒧᔮᒻ ᐅᐦᒋ ᐃᔑᒫᑯᓂᔫ ᐊᓂᔫ ᐅᓂᐯᐅᑲᒥᒄ.

ᓃᔓ ᑑᔥᑌᐤ ᐧᐁᑎᐦᒋᐸᔨᔨᒡ ᐁᒄ ᐅᐦᑖᐧᐄ ᑳ ᐄᑎᑯᑦ, "ᓂᑐᐦᑕ ᒫᒃ. ᑖᐹ ᒋᑲ ᐅᐦᒋ ᐄᒉᐸᔫ ᐁ ᓰᐧᐋᑲᒥᐦᐧᑫᔨᓐ ᐱᔑᒄ ᒥᒄ ᒪᓯᓇᐧᐋᔥᑌᐸᔨᐦᑖᔨᓄ. ᒫᒌ ᓂᑑ ᒋᔅᑯᑕᒫᓯ. ᔮᐸᒡ ᐧᐁᔑᓐ ᒋᑲᒌ ᐃᐦᑑᑌᓐ ᐊᓂᐦᐄᐦ ᑫᐧᑲᔫ ᑳᒌ ᐃᐦᑑᑕᒪᓐ ᑲᔦ ᒥᒄ ᑖᓐ ᐁ ᐃᔑ ᓇᐦᐋᒋᐦᐄᑯᔨᓐ ᑫᐧᑳᓐ ᐁ ᐃᑌᔨᐦᑕᒪᓐ ᒋᐹ ᒥᔦᔨᐦᑌᓐ ᐃᐦᑑᑕᒪᓐ ᒋᑲᒌ ᐃᐦᑑᑌᓐ, ᒥᒄ ᑮᐹ ᓇᒧᐃ ᒋᑲᒌ ᐃᔑᓈᑯᓐ ᐁᑳ ᒌᔑᐦᑖᔨᓄ ᐁ ᒋᔅᑯᑕᒫᓯᔨᓐ ᐊᓂᑌ ᒋᔅᑯᑕᒫᒉᐅᑲᒥᑯᐦᒡ. ᑖᐹ ᒋᑲ ᐴᓈᐸᒥᓰ ᐊᐧᐁᓐ ᐁ ᓰᐧᐋᑲᒥᐦᐧᑫᑦ ᒉᒌ ᐃᑌᔨᐦᑕᐦᒃ ᓰᔅ ᐁᑯᓐ ᐁ ᐃᔅᐧᑳᒡ ᓂᐱᒫᑎᓰᐧᐃᓐ".

ᐊᓂᔫ ᒦᓐ ᐧᐃᔮᐸᓂᔨᒡ ᑳᐤ ᒌ ᓂᑑ ᐲᐦᒉᐤ ᒋᔅᑯᑕᒫᒉᐅᑲᒥᑯᐦᒡ ᑲᔦ ᒦᓐ ᒌ ᒉᑐᐧᐁᒉᐤ ᐅᐧᐄᒉᐧᐋᑲᓐ ᐦᐧᐋᑮ ᐁ ᒥᑐᐧᐁᐧᑖᐤ. ᒌ ᑲᐧᑫᒋᒥᑰ ᒋᔅᑯᑕᒫᒉᐅᑲᒥᒄ ᐅᒋᒫᐤᐦ ᑖᓂᑌ ᑳ ᐃᐦᑖᑦ. ᑳ ᐄᑖᑦ, "ᓂᑐᐦᑯᐃᓂᑲᒥᑯᐦᒡ ᓂᒌ ᐃᑐᐦᑌᓐ ᐁᒄ ᐁ ᐃᐦᑖᔮᐦᒡ ᐱᔑᒄ ᑳ ᐃᐦᑖᔮᓐ", ᒌ ᐃᑌᐤ. ᑳ ᐄᒉᔅᐧᑫᐸᔨᐦᐆᑦ ᐊᓂᔫ ᑳ ᐄᑖᑦ. ᓇᒧᐃ ᐅᐦᒋ ᐧᐄ ᐧᐄᐦᑕᒧᐧᐁᐤ ᐁ ᓰᐧᐋᑲᒥᐦᐧᑫᑦ.

pas à ses entraînements de hockey. Il n'alla pas à ses matchs de hockey. Il ne vit pas de spécialiste du diabète.

hockey games. He didn't see a diabetes specialist.

Au bout d'une semaine, sa chambre commença à sentir un peu le renfermé.

After a week, his bedroom began to smell a bit ripe.

Après deux semaines, son père lui dît : « Écoute. La télévision ne va pas faire disparaître le diabète. Va à l'école. Tu peux toujours faire tout ce que tu faisais avant, tu peux toujours être tout ce que tu veux être, à moins que tu ne finisses pas l'école secondaire. Le diabète n'est pas la fin du monde ».

After two weeks, his dad said, "Look. Television doesn't actually make diabetes go away. Go to school. You can still do everything you did before, you can still be whatever you want to be, unless you don't finish high school. Diabetes isn't the end of the world."

Le lendemain, Jonathan était de retour à l'école et jouait à nouveau au hockey. Le directeur de l'école lui demanda où il était. « Je suis allé à la clinique, puis je suis resté à la maison », dit-il en détournant le regard. Impossible qu'il mentionne *quoi que ce soit* à propos du diabète.

The next day, Jonathan was back in school and playing hockey again. The school principal asked where he'd been. "I went to the clinic and then I stayed home," he said, and looked away. No way was he saying *anything* about diabetes.

ᐊᓂᔮ ᒫᒃ ᑳ ᑎᐧᐃᔥᑖᔨᒡ ᒌᐦ ᓂᑎᐧᐋᐱᒫᐤ
ᐊᓂᔮᐦ ᐊᐧᐋᔨᐤᐦ ᑳ ᐧᐄᒋᐦᐋᔨᒡᐦ ᐊᐧᐋᔨᐤᐦ
ᐋᐦ ᓵᑳᐱᔨᔨᒡᐦ, ᐋᐦ ᔖᐳᒋᔅᒑᔨᐦᑏᒥᔨᒡᐦ
ᐋᐦ ᓵᑳᐅᐱᔨᓈᓂᐧᐃᐧᐃᔨᒡ᙮ ᒌᐦ ᐧᐄᐦᑎᒫᑰ
ᑯᑎᒃᐦ ᐊᐧᐋᔨᐤᐦ ᐧᐄᒋᐦᐄᓯᔨᐤᐦ ᐋᑳ ᓈᔥᒡ
ᒑ ᒌᐦ ᒫᑯᐦᐄᑯᔨᒡᐦ ᐋᐦ ᓵᑳᐅᐱᔨᔨᒡᐦ ᐋᐦ
ᑭᓂᐧᐋᐱᐦᑎᒥᔨᒡᐦ ᐊᓂᔮ ᐋᔑᒦᒋᓯᔨᒡᐦ ᑭᔮᐦ
ᐊᑎᑎᐤ ᐋᐦ ᔖᔖᐧᐃᔨᒡᐦ, ᒥᒄ ᒫᒃ ᐧᐄᔨ
ᐧᒑᓂᑫᓐ ᓂᑐᐦᑯᔨᓐᐦ ᑭᑎ ᐋᐱᒋᐦᑖᐤ ᑭᔮᐦ ᒫᒃ
ᐄᓐᓯᓚᓐ, ᑭᔮᐦ ᒑᑳᑦ ᒥᓯᐧᐋ ᐊᐧᐋᓂᒌ ᐱᑎᒫ
ᒥᒄ ᓂᑐᐦᑯᔨᓐᐦ ᐋᐱᒋᐦᑖᐧᐃᒡ᙮ ᐊᓂᑖᐦ ᐲᐦᒋᔨᐤ
ᐋᑯᑖᐦ ᐋᐦ ᐃᐦᑎᑯᐦᒡ ᐅᐲᔥᐲᔥᒃ ᐄᔑᓂᐦᑳᑖᐤ,
ᐋᑯᑎᐦ ᐊᓂᑎᐦ ᐧᐋᔑᐦᑖᒐᐱᔨᒡ ᐄᓐᓯᓚᓐ,
ᐋᔪᐧᐃᒄ ᒫᒃ ᓂᒥ ᐄᔥᐱᔑ ᐅᔑᐦᑖᒐᐱᔨᔨᐤ
ᐧᒑᓂᑫᓐ ᐅᔮᐦᒡ ᑭᔮᐦ ᓂᑐᐦᑯᔨᓐᐦ ᐋᐱᒋᐦᑖᒐ
ᐊᑎᑎᐤ ᓈᔥᒡ ᒥᔥᑏᐦ ᒐ ᐋᐱᑎᓰᒥᑭᓂᔨᒡ ᐊᓂᔮ
ᐅᐲᔥᐲᔥᒃᐦ ᐄᓐᓯᓚᓐ ᐋᐦ ᐅᔥᑖᒐᐱᔨᔨᒡ᙮ ᒐᒃ
ᒫᒃ ᐊᑐᒡ ᓈᔥᑎᔨᒡ ᒌᐦᐄᓂᔨᐤ, ᐄᑎᑰ, ᐋᑯᑎᐦ
ᒫᒃ ᐊᓂᑎᐦ ᐋᔑᓈᑯᓂᔨᒡ ᒑ ᒌᐦ ᒌᔥᑎᐦᐅᓯᒡ
ᐊᐧᐋᓂᒌ ᒑ ᒌᐦ ᒥᔨᓯᒡ ᐄᓐᓯᓚᓐ᙮

"ᓂᒧᐃ ᐋ ᐊᑎᑎᐤ ᐱᒥᐧᔮᐤ", ᐄᔑ ᑯᐧᑳᒋᒫᐤ
ᐧᒑᓂᑫᓐ, "ᐋᑳ ᐅᑎᓂᒫᓐ ᓂᑐᐦᑯᔨᓐᐦ ᒥᒄ
ᐄᓐᓯᓚᓐ ᐋᐱᒋᐦᑖᔮᓐ᙮ ᐊᑐᒡ ᓈᔥᒡ ᒥᔥᑏᐦ
ᐋᐱᑎᓰᒥᑭᓐ ᐊᓐ ᓂᐲᔥᐲᔥᒃ᙮"

"ᐄᐦᐄ," ᐄᑎᑰ, "ᒥᒄ ᒫᒃ ᒋᒋᔅᒑᔨᐦᑖᓐ ᐋ ᑖᓐ
ᑎᐦᐧᑖᐤ ᒋᐱᐦ ᒌᔥᑎᐦᐅᓯᓐ᙮"

ᒌᐦ ᐄᔨᑮᔮᔮᐦᑎᒻ ᐧᒑᓂᑫᓐ ᐊᓂᔮ ᑳ ᐄᔑ
ᒥᒫᑎᐧᐋᑦ ᐋᐦ ᐧᐋᐧᐋᐹᔅᑯᐦᐄᒑᓂᐧᐃᐧᐃᔨᒡ
ᐋᐦ ᐱᔥᑎᐦᐅᑯᑦ ᐊᓂᔮᐦ ᑳ ᐧᐋᐧᐋᔮᓯᔨᒡᐦ,

ᐊᓂᔫ ᑳ ᑑᔥᑌᔨᒡ ᒌ ᓂᑐᐧᐋᐸᒣᐤ ᐊᓂᔫ
ᓂᑐᐦᑯᐃᓂᔅᐧᑫᐤ ᑳ ᓰᐧᐋᑲᒥᐦᐧᑫᔨᐧᑖᐤ ᑳ
ᓇᓈᑲᒋᐦᐋᔨᒡ᙮ ᑳ ᐃᑎᑯᑦ ᐸᔅᒡ ᐊᐧᐁᓂᒌ ᐁ
ᑲᔅᒋᐦᐅᐧᑖᐤ ᐁ ᒦᓇᐱᑕᐦᐧᑳᐤ ᐁ ᓰᐧᐋᑲᒥᐦᐧᑫᐧᑖᐤ
ᐁ ᓇᓈᑲᒋᐦᑖᐧᑖᐤ ᐁ ᐃᔑ ᒦᒋᓱᐧᑖᐤ ᑲᔦ ᐁᑎᑑ
ᐁ ᐋᔫᐦᒌᐧᑖᐤ, ᒥᒄ ᒫᒃ ᒌ ᐃᑎᑰ ᒉ ᐅᑎᓇᐦᒃ
ᓂᑐᐦᑯᐃᓐᐦ ᒫᒃ ᐃᓐᓯᓚᓐ ᒉ ᐅᑎᓇᐦᒃ ᐧᐄᔭ,
ᑯᑕᑲᒡ ᐊᐧᐁᓂᒌ ᓃᔥᑕᒻ ᓂᑐᐦᑯᐃᓐᐦ ᐅᑎᓇᒧᒡ᙮
ᐧᐄᔭ ᒫᒃ ᐃᓐᓯᓚᓐ ᒌ ᓂᑐᐧᐁᔨᐦᑖᑯᓂᔫ
ᑫᒌ ᐅᑎᓇᐦᒃ, ᐅᐦᐹᐱᑯᓰᐦᒡ ᐊᐧᐁᓐ ᐁᑯᑌ
ᐧᐁᐦᒋ ᐅᔑᐦᑖᒉᐸᔨᐦᒡ ᐃᓐᓯᓚᓐ ᐁᒄ ᒫᒃ
ᒥᒄ ᓂᑐᐦᑯᐃᓐ ᐅᑎᓇᐦᑫ ᐁᑎᑑ ᓰᐦᒃ ᒋᐹ
ᐋᐸᑎᓰᒪᑲᓂᔫ ᐅᐦᐹᐱᑯᓰᒻ᙮ ᒋᐹ ᐃᔑᓈᑯᓂᔫ
ᑫᒃ ᐁᑳ ᒥᒍᓐ ᓵᐱᓰᒪᑲᓂᔨᒡ᙮ ᐁᐅᒄ ᐅᔫ ᑳ
ᐃᔑ ᐧᐋᐧᐄᐦᑕᒫᑯᑦ᙮ ᑲᔦ ᒌ ᐄᑎᑰ, ᐊᐧᐁᓐ
ᐁᑳ ᓵᔅ ᓵᐲᒪᑲᓂᔨᒡ ᐅᐦᐹᐱᑯᓰᒻ ᐁᑯᑦ
ᓄᑐᐧᐁᔨᐦᑖᑯᓂᔨᒡ ᒉᒌ ᐸᒋᔅᑲᐦᐆᓱᑦ᙮

ᑳ ᐄᑖᑦ ᐊᓂᔫ ᓂᑐᐦᑯᐃᓂᔅᐧᑫᐤ, "ᓇᒧᐃ
ᐋ ᒫᒃ ᓂᐹᒌ ᐸᒋᔅᑲᐦᐆᓱᓐ, ᐁᑳ ᐅᑎᓇᒫᓐ
ᐊᓂᔫ ᓂᑐᐦᑯᐃᓐᐦ᙮ ᓇᒧᐃ ᒋᐹ ᐅᐦᒋ ᐃᔥᐱᔥ
ᐋᐸᑎᓰᒪᑲᓐ ᓂᐹᐦᐱᑯᓰᒻ ᐊᓐ ᐃᐦᑎᔮᓄ᙮"

"ᐁᐦᐁ", ᒌ ᐄᑎᑰ, "ᒋᒋᔅᑫᔨᐦᑌᓐ ᐋ ᒫᒃ ᑕᐦᑐ
ᐸᒋᔥᑲᐦᐄᑲᓐ ᑫ ᐋᐸᒋᐦᑖᔭᓐ"᙮

ᒌ ᒋᔅᑫᔨᐦᑕᒻ ᑖᓐ ᐁ ᐃᑌᔨᐦᑖᑯᓂᔨᒡ ᐸᒃᐦ
ᐁ ᑖᐅᐦᐆᑯᑦ ᐦᐋᑮ ᐁ ᒣᑐᐧᐁᑦ ᐊᔦ ᐁ
ᑯᒋᔥᑯᐧᐋᑲᓈᑦ ᓄᔅᑕ ᐅᔥᑎᐧᑳᓂᐦᒡ ᐁ ᑖᐅᔑᓂᑦ

Cette semaine-là, il alla également voir un spécialiste du diabète. Elle lui indiqua que certaines personnes pouvaient ultimement contrôler leur diabète en changeant leur régime alimentaire et en faisant plus d'exercice. Toutefois, pour le moment, Jonathan devrait prendre soit des pilules, soit de l'insuline; la plupart des gens commençaient avec des pilules. Son corps avait besoin de plus d'insuline. L'insuline est fabriquée dans le pancréas et les pilules feraient travailler le pancréas plus fort. Il finirait par s'épuiser, dit-elle, et l'épuisement du pancréas est le moment où les gens commencent habituellement à s'injecter de l'insuline avec des seringues.

He went to a diabetes specialist that week too. She said that some people can eventually control diabetes by changing their diet and increasing exercise, but for now Jonathan would have to take either pills or insulin, and most people started with pills. His body needed more insulin, insulin is made in the pancreas, and pills would make the pancreas work harder. Eventually it would burn out, she said, and pancreas burnout is when people usually start injecting insulin with needles.

« Ne serait-il pas plus logique, demanda Jonathan, que je saute les pilules et que je m'injecte simplement de l'insuline ? Je permettrais à mon pancréas de se reposer ».

"Wouldn't it make more sense," Jonathan asked, "if I skipped pills and just injected insulin? I'd be giving my pancreas a break."

« Oui, dit-elle, mais sais-tu combien d'injections cela représentera ? »

"Yes," she said, "but do you know how many needles that will be?"

Jonathan était habitué aux palets volants, aux plaquages, aux commotions, aux membres cassés et aux contusions. Il

Jonathan was used to flying pucks, body checks, concussions, broken limbs, and bruises. He was the enforcer on his

ᐋᐦ ᒍᐦᑯᔥᑭᐧᐋᑭᓂᐧᐃᑦ, ᐅᔥᑎᐧᑳᓂᐦᒡ ᐋᐦ ᐋᑯᐦᐋᑭᓂᐧᐃᑦ, ᐋᐦ ᓈᐧᑖᐲᔨᔨᒡᐦ ᐅᔅᑭᓐᐦ, ᑭᔮᐦ ᐋᐦ ᐅᑐᒋᓯᑦ ᒫᓐᐦ ᐅᐦᒋ ᐊᓂᔮ ᐋᐦ ᒫᐦᑎᐧᐋᑦ᙮ ᐋᐅᒄ ᐧᐋᔥ ᐧᐄᔨ ᑳ ᒌ ᐄᑖᐱᒋᐦᐋᑭᓂᐧᐃᑦ ᐋᐦ ᒫᓯᐦᒑᑦ ᐊᓂᑖᐦ ᒥᔮᑎᐧᐋᐧᑖᐤᐦ᙮ ᐋᔪᐧᐃᒄ ᑳ ᒌ ᐄᑖᐱᑎᔫᑦ ᐋᐦ ᒍᐦᑯᔥᑳᒋᒑᑦ, ᑭᔮᐦ ᐅᔥᑦ ᐋᐦ ᐧᐄᐦ ᒋᔑᐧᐋᐦᐋᑦ ᐊᓂᔮᐦ ᑳ ᒍᒋᐦᐋᒡ ᐊᓂᑎᐦ ᐅᐦᒋ ᒑ ᒌᐦ ᐧᐃᓂᔨᐦᑎᔨᒡᐦ᙮ ᓂᒧᐃ ᐧᐄᔮᔥ ᒋᑭ ᒌᐦ ᐃᐦᑐᑖᑰ ᒥᐦᒑᐧᑖᐤ ᐋᐦ ᒌᔥᑎᐦᐅᔫᑦ ᐹᔨᑯᒌᔑᑳᐤᐦ᙮ ᐋᑳ ᑭᔨᐧᐹ ᒥᒄ ᐧᐋᐱᒥᑯᒑ ᐊᐧᐋᔨᐤᐦ ᐋᐦ ᒌᔥᑎᐦᐅᔫᑦ᙮

ᐋᔪᐧᐃᒄ ᑭᔮᐦ ᑳ ᑯᒋᔥᑖᑦ ᐧᒑᓂᕋᓐ ᐊᑎᑎᐤ ᑯᐃᔅᒄ ᒑ ᒌᐦ ᒦᒋᓯᑦ = ᐋᑳ ᓈᔥᒡ ᒑ ᒦᒋᑦ ᒑᐧᑳᔨᐤ ᒥᔥᑏᐦ ᐋᐦ ᐄᐦᑎᑯᓂᔨᒡ ᓵᑳᔨᐤ, ᓂᑎᐧᐄ ᒑᐧᑳᔨᐤ ᐋᑳ ᒑ ᐧᐄᒋᐦᐄᑯᑦ ᐅᔮᐦᒡ, ᐋᑳ ᒨᔥ ᒑ ᓯᓈᑭᐧᐃᑦ = ᑭᔮᐦ ᒌᐦ ᒌᔥᑎᐦᐅᔫ ᑯᐃᔅᒄ, ᐋᔑᑯᒻ ᒫᒋᔫᒡᐦ ᑭᔮᐦ ᐹᔨᐧᑳᐤ ᐋᐦᐧᒫᔮᐦ ᑭᐧᐃᔑᒧᑦ᙮ ᒑᒃ ᒫᒃ ᒥᒄ ᐋᐱᐦᑎᐤ ᒌᔥᐱᔑ ᓂᑎᐧᐋᔨᐦᑎᒻ ᐄᓐᓯᓚᓐ ᑭᔮᐦ ᐊᓂᑖᐦ ᐄᔑ ᐹᔨᑯᐲᓯᒻ ᐄᔑ ᓃᔥᑖᒥᐦᒡ ᒦᓐ ᐊᑎᑎᐤ ᓂᒥ ᐅᐦᒋ ᓂᑎᐧᐋᔨᐦᑎᒻ᙮ ᒑᒃ ᓈᔥᑎᔨᒡ ᓂᒥ ᐅᐦᒋ ᐋᐱᒋᐦᑖᐤ ᐄᓐᓯᓚᓐ ᑭᔮᐦ ᐊᓂᔮᐦ ᓂᑐᐦᑯᔨᓐᐦ ᑳ ᒥᔮᑭᓂᐧᐃᑦ᙮ ᓈᔥᒡ ᐋᐦ ᒌᐦ ᒥᔪᐱᔨᑦ: ᓈᔥᒡ ᒥᔥᑏᐦ ᓃᐦᑖᐦᒡ ᐋᐦ ᒌᐦ ᐄᔅᐱᔨᔨᒡ ᐊᓂᔮ ᐋᐦ ᓵᑳᐅᐱᔨᔨᑦ᙮ ᒥᒄ ᒫᒃ ᐋᔨᐱᒡ ᓂᒥ ᐅᐦᒋ ᐧᐄᐦᑎᒧᐧᐋᐤ ᐊᐧᐋᔨᐤᐦ ᐊᓂᔮ ᐋᐦ ᓵᑳᐅᐱᔨᑦ᙮

ᑲᔦ ᐁ ᓈᐧᑖᐦᑕᑖᑦ ᐅᔅᑲᓐ ᑲᔦ ᒫᒃ ᐁ ᐧᐊᑑᑲᐦᐆᐧᐋᑲᓈᑦ᙮ ᐧᐃ ᒫᐅᒡ ᒌ ᐋᐦᐧᑳᑌᔨᐦᑖᑯᓰ ᐁ ᒣᑐᐧᐁᐧᑖᐤ ᐅᐧᐄᒋᒣᑐᐧᐁᓰᒻᐦ᙮ ᒫᔅᑫᓰ ᒌ ᐄᑖᐸᒋᐦᐋᑲᓈ ᐊᓂᔫᐦ ᒣᑐᐧᐁᓰᐦ ᑳ ᑯᒋᐦᐊᐧᑖᐤ ᐁ ᒫᓯᐦᐋᑦ ᒫᒃ ᑫᐧᑳᔫ ᐁ ᐃᐦᑑᑕᐧᐋᑦ ᑫᒌ ᐅᐦᒋ ᒋᔑᐧᐋᓯᔨᒡ᙮ ᓇᒧᐃ ᒫᒃ ᐧᐃᔦᔅ ᒋᐹ ᐅᐦᒋ ᐃᑌᔨᐦᑕᒻ ᐸᒋᔥᑲᐦᐆᓯᑦ ᒣᓯᑯᒻ ᒌᔑᑳᐤ᙮ ᑌᐱᔮᐦᒡ ᐁᑳ ᐧᐋᐸᒥᑦ ᐊᐧᐁᓐ, ᒌ ᐃᑌᔨᐦᑕᒻ᙮

ᒌ ᒋᐦ ᒋᐸᔨᐦᑖᐤ ᑯᐃᔅᒄ ᐁ ᐃᔑ ᒦᒋᓯᑦ = ᐊᐱᔔᔥ ᒥᒄ ᐸᐦᐧᑫᔑᑲᓂᐦᒡ ᑳ ᐃᑌᔨᐦᑖᑯᓂᔨᒡ ᒦᒋᒥᔫ ᒌ ᒦᒎ, ᓇᒧᐃ ᓈᔅᒡ ᐅᐦᒋ ᒦᒍ ᐁᑳ ᒥᔫᔅᑳᑫᔨᒡ ᒦᒋᒥᔫ, ᓇᒧᐃ ᐅᐦᒋ ᐃᔥᐱᔥ ᓯᓈᑭᔫ = ᒨᔥ ᒌ ᐅᑎᓇᒻ ᐅᓂᑐᐦᑯᐃᓈᐳᓐ ᑖᐦᐧᑖᐤ ᒋᐹ ᐅᑎᓇᒻ, ᒌ ᐸᒋᔅᑲᐦᐆᔫ ᑕᐦᐧᑖᐤ ᒫᒋᓯᒡ ᑲᔦ ᑫ ᐊᑎ ᑰᔑᒧᒡ᙮ ᐁᑎᑑ ᓰᒃ ᒌ ᔅᓵᐧᐁᔫ ᑖᓐ ᑳ ᐯᒋ ᐃᐦᑎᑦ ᐊᓂᑌ ᐅᑖᐦᒡ᙮ ᓇᒧᐃ ᒥᐦᑫᑐ ᐲᓯᒻᐦ ᑫᒃ ᒥᒄ ᐋᐱᐦᑑ ᒌ ᐃᔥᐱᔥ ᐅᑎᓇᒻ ᐊᓂᔫ ᐅᓂᑐᐦᑯᐃᓈᐳᒻ ᐁᒄ ᒦᓐ ᐯᔨᒄ ᐲᓯᒻ ᐊᓂᑌ ᐃᔑ ᔩᐸᒡ ᒦᓐ ᐊᐱᐦᑑ ᐊᓂᔫ ᑳ ᐃᔥᐱᔥ ᐅᑎᓇᐦᒃ ᒌ ᐅᑎᓇᒻ᙮ ᑫᒃ ᓇᒧᐃ ᐅᐦᒋ ᓂᑐᐧᐁᔨᐦᑕᒻ ᑲᔦ ᐊᓂᔫ ᐅᓂᑐᐦᑯᐃᓂᒻᐦ ᑳᒌ ᐅᑎᐦᐊᒃ ᐊᐧᐁᓐ ᐁ ᔫᐧᐋᑲᒥᐦᐧᑫᑦ ᓇᒧᐃ ᐅᐦᒋ ᓂᑐᐧᐁᔨᐦᑕᒻ᙮ ᐊᓂᔫ ᐁᒌ ᒥᔫᓈᓈᑲᒋᐦᐄᓯᑦ ᐧᐁᐅᒄ ᐧᐁᐦᒌ ᐁᑳ ᓂᑐᐧᐁᔨᐦᑕᐦᒃ ᓰᔅ ᐊᓂᔫᐦ ᓂᑐᐦᑯᐃᓐᐦ = ᒥᒍᓐ ᐧᐃᔨ ᐁᒌ ᒫᔑᐦᑖᑦ ᐁᑳ ᑫᒌ ᑎᐯᔨᒥᑯᑦ ᒋᐦᒋᐧᐁ ᒫᒃ ᒥᔅᑕᐦᐄ ᐁᒌ ᔫᐧᐋᑲᒥᐦᐧᑫᑦ᙮ ᔩᐸᒡ ᒫᒃ ᓇᒧᐃ ᐧᐋᒋ ᐯᔨᒄ ᐊᐧᐁᔫᐦ ᐅᐦᒋ ᐧᐄᐦᑕᒧᐧᐁᐤ ᐁᒌ ᐊᔩᑦ ᐅᔫ ᐋᐦᑯᓯᐧᐃᓂᔫ᙮

était l'homme fort de son équipe de hockey, le goon. Son travail consistait à s'occuper des coups sur la glace et même à essayer d'énerver les joueurs de l'autre équipe pour leur faire rater leur coup. Tout un tas de petites aiguilles chaque jour ne serait pas un problème. Aussi longtemps que personne ne les voyait.

hockey team, the goon. His job was to do the hitting on the ice, and even to try to aggravate players on the other team and make them screw up. A bunch of little needles every day were not a big deal. As long as no one saw them.

Jonathan commença à manger plus prudemment – moins de glucides, moins de malbouffe, des collations moins fréquentes – et il prenait son insuline religieusement : une injection chaque fois qu'il mangeait et une autre avant de se coucher. Il s'entraînait encore plus qu'avant. Après quelques mois, il avait seulement besoin d'environ la moitié de son insuline et un mois plus tard, la moitié de celle-ci. Bientôt, il ne prenait plus du tout d'insuline ni de médicaments contre le diabète. Il avait fait d'importants progrès : il avait maîtrisé son diabète grave. Toutefois, il ne dit toujours à personne qu'il avait la maladie.

Jonathan began to eat more carefully – fewer carbohydrates, less junk food, less frequent snacking – and took his insulin religiously, one shot every time he ate and another before bed. He worked out even more than he had before. After a few months, he needed about half as much insulin and another month later, half of that. Soon he wasn't using insulin or any diabetes medication at all. He had made important progress: he had brought severe diabetes under control. But he still didn't tell anyone that he had the disease.

ᓂᒧᐃ ᓈᔥᑎᔨᒡ ᓂᓂᑎᐧᐋᔨᒫᐤ ᐊᐧᐋᓐ ᒑ ᒋᔅᒑᐊᔨᐦᑎᐦᒃ ᐋᐦ ᔖᑳᐅᐱᔨᔮᓐ, ᐄᑖᔨᐦᑎᒻ ᒫᐧᑳᒡ ᐋᐦ ᑯᐧᑳᑖᐧᐄᑦ᙮ ᑯᔥᑖᑎᑯᓂᔨᐤ ᐋᐦ ᐧᐄᐦᑎᒧᐧᐋᑭᓂᐅᐧᐃᒡ ᐊᐧᐋᓂᒌ, ᐄᑖᔨᐦᑎᒻ, ᒫᐧᑳᒡ ᓰᐦᒃ ᐋᐦ ᑯᒋᔥᑖᑦ ᒑ ᒌᐦ ᐅᐦᐱᓃᓯᑦ ᐊᑎᑎᐤ ᒑ ᒌᐦ ᒥᔥᑎᐧᐄᑦ᙮ ᐋᑦ ᒥᒄ ᓈᔥᒡ ᐊᐱᔒᔥ ᐄᔨᐦᒡ ᐄᑖᔨᐦᑖᑯᓯᑦ ᐊᐧᐋᓐ ᐊᓂᑖᐦ ᒋᔅᑯᑎᒫᑑᑭᒥᑯᐦᒡ ᐊᔮᐱᐤ ᓈᔥᒡ ᒎᔥ ᒥᒫᔮᔨᒫᑭᓂᐆ᙮ ᐧᒫᐦᒡ ᐊᓐ ᐃᔥᐧᑳᔑᔥ ᐋᑦ ᒥᒄ ᐊᐱᔒᔥ ᒌᐦ ᒥᓯᓂᐦᐅᓯᑦ ᐅᔥᒌᔑᒄ ᐊᔮᐱᐤ ᓈᔥᒡ ᒌᐦ ᒫᒫᐦᒌᔨᑖᑭᓂᐆ᙮ ᐊᓂᔮᐦ ᒫᒃ ᒫᐅᒡ ᑳ ᐧᐄᐦ ᓂᓈᐹᐧᐃᔨᒡᐦ ᓈᐹᔑᔥᐦ ᐊᓂᑖᐦ ᒋᔅᑯᑎᒫᑑᑭᒥᑯᐦᒡ ᒎᔥ ᒌᐦ ᐧᐄᐦ ᒫᔑᐦᐄᑰ ᐧᒑᓂᓕᓐ ᐋᔫᐧᐃᒄ ᐋᑯᐦ ᐊᓂᔮ ᐄᔨᔨᐦᒡ ᐋᐦ ᐄᑎᔅᑳᓈᓯᑦ ᑭᔮᐦ ᐋᐱᐦᑎᐤ ᐋᐦ ᒌᐦ ᐧᐋᒥᔥᑎᑯᔒᐧᐃᑦ᙮ ᒥᔑᐤ ᒋᔅᒑᐦᑎᑭᓂᐧᐃᒑ ᐋᐦ ᔖᑳᐅᐱᔨᔨᔮᓐ, ᓂᒧᐃ ᓈᓂᑎᐤ ᓂᑭ ᒌᐦ ᒌᐧᐋᓐ, ᐄᑖᔨᐦᑎᒻ ᒫᐧᑳᒡ ᓈᔥᒡ ᓰᐦᒃ ᐋᐦ ᑯᐧᑳᑖᐧᐄᑦ᙮

ᐹᔨᐧᑳᐤ ᐋᐦ ᒌᔑᑳᔨᒡ ᐊᓂᑖᐦ ᒋᔅᑯᑎᒫᑑᑭᒥᑯᐦᒡ, ᐊᓂᑖᐦ ᐋᐦ ᒋᔥᑖᐹᐧᐄᓈᓂᐧᐃᔨᒡ ᐋᐦ ᓃᐳᐧᐃᑦ ᐧᒑᓂᓕᓐ᙮ ᐱᔮᒋ ᐋᐱᐦᐄᐱᔨᔨᒡᐦ ᒋᔥᑐᐦᑭᓐᐦ, ᐱᔮᒋᐲᐦᒋᒑᔨᒡᐦ ᐊᓂᔮᐦ ᒫᐅᒡ ᑳ ᐧᐄᐦ ᓂᓈᐹᐧᐄᒡᐦ ᓈᐹᔑᔥᐦ ᑭᔮᐦ ᐱᔮᒋᓈᑖᑦ ᐧᒑᓂᓕᓐᐦ ᔖᔥ ᑭᔨᐧᐹ ᒥᐦᒑᐧᑖᐤ ᐊᓂᑖᐦ ᐋᐦ ᒌᐦ ᐃᐦᑐᑎᐧᐋᑦ᙮ ᐧᐋᒥᔥᑎᑯᔒᐤ, ᐄᑎᑰ, ᑭᔮᐦ ᑖᐦᒋᔥᑳᑯᑦ ᐅᑎᒋᔒᐦᒡ ᐅᐦᒋᑯᓂᔨᐤ ᐋᐦ ᐋᐱᒋᐦᑖᔨᒡᐦ᙮

ᓂᒥᒌᔨᐧᐋ ᒋᔅᒋᓰ ᑖᓐ ᐋᔥᐱᔑ ᒋᔑᐧᐋᐦᐄᑯᑦ ᐊᓂᔮᐦ ᑳ ᐧᐄᐦᓂᓈᐹᐧᐃᔨᒡᐦ, ᑭᔮᐦ ᓂᒥᒌᔨᐧᐋ ᒋᔅᒋᔫᑎᑎᒻ ᐊᓂᔮ ᐋᐦ ᔖᑳᐅᐱᔨᑦ, ᑭᔮᐦ ᑖᓐ ᐋᔥᐱᔑ ᔖᔥ ᒥᔥᑭᐧᐄᑦ ᑳ ᐄᔥᐱᔑ ᒎᔥ

ᓇᒧᐃ ᐊᐧᐁᓐ ᑲᑕᒌ ᒋᔅᒉᔨᐦᑕᒻ, ᒌ ᐃᑌᔨᐦᑕᒻ ᒣᐧᑳᒡ ᐁ ᐅᐦᐱᓂᒉᑦ᙮ ᑯᔥᑖᑎᑯᓐ ᐁ ᐧᐄᐦᑕᒧᐧᐋᑲᓈᐧᑖᐤ ᐊᐧᐁᓂᒌ, ᒌ ᐃᑎᓰ ᐁ ᐊᑎ ᐅᐦᐱᐸᔨᐦᐄᓯᑦ ᐅᐧᑳᐦᑯᓄᒻ ᐁ ᑖᐦᒋᔑᒫᑦ ᐊᓂᑕ ᐊᓂᔫ ᐱᐧᔮᐱᔅᑯᔫ ᑳ ᐱᒥᑖᔅᑯᓂᔨᒡ᙮ ᐧᐁᔅ ᐊᓂᑌ ᒋᔅᑯᑕᒫᑑᑲᒥᑯᐦᒡ ᒎᔥ ᒫᓴᔨᒫᑲᓅ ᐊᐧᐁᓐ ᐊᐱᔒᔥ ᐋᐦᒌᐤᐦ ᐁ ᐃᑌᔨᐦᑖᑯᓯᑦ᙮ ᒧᐧᐁᐦᒡ ᐊᓐ ᐃᔅᐧᑫᔥ ᐋᑦ ᒥᒄ ᐊᐱᔒᔥ ᐁ ᒌ ᐧᐊᐧᐁᔑᐦᐅᑦ ᓂᑕᒧᒄ ᒌ ᐃᔑᓂᐦᑳᑖᑲᓅ ᐁ ᒫᓴᔨᒫᑲᓅᑦ᙮ ᑲᓴ ᒫᒃ ᐊᓐ ᓈᐯᔥ ᒫᐅᒡ ᑳ ᓰᐦᒋᓰᑦ ᑳ ᐃᑌᔨᒫᑲᓅᑦ ᐊᓂᑌ ᒋᔅᑯᑕᒫᒉᐅᑲᒥᑯᐦᒡ ᓵᔅ ᐁᑯᓐ ᑳ ᐃᐦᑐᑕᐧᐋᑦ ᐧᒑᓇᓓᓐ ᐁ ᒪᒫᔑᐦᐋᑦ ᒥᒄ ᐊᓂᔫ ᐋᐱᐦᑑ ᐄᓅ ᐁ ᐃᐦᑖᔨᒡ, ᐋᐱᐦᑑ ᐧᐁᒥᔅᑎᑰᔫᐤ ᐁ ᐃᐦᑖᑦ᙮ ᒋᔅᒉᔨᐦᑕᐦᐧᑳᐧᐁᓂᒡ ᐁ ᔫᐧᐋᑲᒥᐦᐧᑫᐅᒡ ᓇᒧᐃ ᓈᓂᑑ ᓂᑲ ᐅᐦᒋ ᐅᑎᐦᑌᓐ ᓃᒋᓈᓐ, ᒌ ᐃᑌᔨᐦᑕᒻ ᒣᐧᑳᒡ ᒥᔅᑳᑦ ᓴᓵᐅᐸᔨᓈᐧᐋᑲᓂᔫ ᐁ ᐋᐸᒋᐦᑖᑦ᙮

ᐯᔨᐧᑳᐤ ᐊᓂᑌ ᒋᔅᑯᑕᒫᒉᐅᑲᒥᑯᐦᒡ ᐁ ᐃᐦᑖᑦ, ᒦᔫᐅᑲᒥᑯᐦᒡ ᒌ ᐲᐦᑫᐤ ᐁᒄ ᑳ ᓃᐳᑦ ᐯᔕᒡ ᐊᓂᑕ ᑲᒌ ᒋᔅᑖᐸᐅᑎᐦᒑᓄᔨᒡ᙮ ᑳ ᐅᐦᒋ ᐋᐸᐦᐄᐸᔨᔨᒡ ᒋᔅᑐᐦᑲᓐ ᐧᐁᐦᒋ ᐲᐦᑫᔨᐦᒡ ᐊᓂᔫ ᒫᐅᒡ ᑳ ᑯᔥᑖᑎᑯᓯᔨᒡ ᓈᐯᔅ ᐊᓂᑕ ᒋᔅᑯᑕᒫᒉᐅᑲᒥᑯᐦᒡ ᒌᐧᐁᐦᒡ ᓂᔨᑎᑯᑦ ᐊᓂᔫ ᐹᐦᑫᔨᒡ ᐁᐅᒄ ᑮᐹ ᑲᒌ ᐃᐦᑑᑖᑯᑦ ᒫᓐᐦ ᐊᓂᔫ ᓈᐯᔅ᙮ "ᐧᐁᒥᔅᑎᑰᔫᐤ", ᒌ ᐄᑎᑰ ᐁ ᒫᓴᔨᒥᑯᑦ ᐁᒄ ᑳ ᑯᒋᔥᑳᑯᑦ ᓇᐦᐋᐤ ᐅᔅᑲᑖᐦᒡ ᐅᐦᒋᑯᓐ ᐁ ᐋᐸᒋᐦᑖᔨᒡ᙮

ᓇᒧᐃ ᒉᒋᒻ ᐅᐦᒌ ᒫᒥᑐᓀᔨᐦᑕᒻ ᐱᑕᒫ ᑖᓐ ᐁ ᐃᔥᐱᔥ ᓯᔅᑲᒋᐦᐄᑯᑦ ᐊᓂᔫ ᐁ ᐃᐦᑑᑖᑯᑦ ᑲᓴ ᐊᓂᔫ ᐁ ᔫᐧᐋᑲᒥᐦᐧᑫᑦ ᐁᑲ ᓂᑐᐧᐁᔨᒫᑦ ᑯᑕᒃ ᐊᐧᐁᔫ ᒉᒌ ᒋᔅᒉᔨᐦᑕᒥᔨᒡ,

Il faut que ce soit un secret, se disait-il en poussant sur la barre de poids. *C'est dangereux de le dire aux gens*, pensait-il, en hissant son menton au-dessus de la barre de traction. Toute personne à l'école qui était un tant soit peu différente était intimidée régulièrement. Comme cette fille qui s'était fait harceler et traitée d'agace juste parce qu'elle avait porté un peu de maquillage pour les yeux. Le gars le plus tough de l'école battait déjà Jonathan parce qu'il était à moitié Cri, à moitié blanc. *S'ils découvrent que je suis aussi diabétique, je ne rentrerai jamais à la maison*, pensait-il, en forçant contre les plaques de la machine à jambes.

It has to be secret, he said to himself as he bench-pressed the barbell. *It's dangerous to tell people,* he thought, hoisting his chin over the chin-up bar. Anybody at school who was a little bit different was bullied regularly. Like that girl who got harassed and called a slut just because she wore a bit of eye makeup. The toughest guy in school was already beating Jonathan up for being half-Cree, half-white. *If they find out I'm diabetic too, I'll never make it home,* he thought, straining against the plates on the leg machine.

Un jour, à l'école, Jonathan se tenait devant le lavabo dans la salle de bains. La porte s'ouvrit brutalement et le gars le plus tough de l'école s'en prit à Jonathan comme il l'avait fait tant de fois auparavant. « sale blanc », railla-t-il et il lui donna un coup de genou dans le ventre.

At school one day, Jonathan stood at the sink in the bathroom. The door swung open and the toughest guy in school walked in and came at Jonathan as he had so many times before. "White boy" he jeered, and kneed him in the stomach.

Jonathan ne pensa pas à la frustration qu'il ressentait à l'égard du gros dur, ni à son secret concernant le diabète, ni à quel point tous ses exercices supplémentaires

Jonathan didn't think about how frustrated he was with the tough guy, nor about his diabetes secret, nor about how much stronger all the extra workouts had

ᑯᐧᑳᑖᐧᐄᑦ᙮ ᒥᒄ ᐋᔥᐱᔒᑦ ᐧᐋᑖᒧᐦᐧᐋᑦ ᐊᓂᑎᐦ ᐅᔅᑭᐦᑎᑯᔪᒡᐦ᙮ ᓈᐧᐋᐱᔪᑦ ᐊᓐ ᓈᐹᔑᔥ ᑭᔫᐦ ᐊᓂᑖᐦ ᓂᐱᒋᔅᑎᑯᐦᒡ ᐋᔑ ᐱᐦᒋᔑᐦᒃ᙮ ᐋᑯᑎᐦ ᐹᒥᔑᐦᒃ ᐧᐋᔪᐱᔥᒌᔥ, ᒑᒃ ᐧᐋᓂᔥᑳᑦ ᑭᔫᐦ ᓂᒥ ᓂᐦᑖ ᒦᓐ ᐅᐦᒋ ᐱᒫᔪᒥᑰ ᐧᒑᓂᓀᓐ᙮ ᓂᒥ ᓰᐦᒃ ᓈᐅᔥ ᐊᓂᑖᐦ ᒋᔅᑯᑎᒫᑑᑭᒥᑯᐦᒡ ᑳᐦ ᒋᔅᑯᑎᒫᒑᓂᐧᐃᒡ ᐋᐦ ᐃᐦᑐᑖᑯᒡ ᐊᐧᐋᓂᒌ ᓈᔥᒡ ᐋᐦ ᐧᐄᐦ ᒥᒫᔫᔪᒫᑭᓂᐅᐧᐃᒡ᙮ ᐋᑯᑎᐦ ᒫᒃ ᐄᔪᐦᒡ ᑳ ᐅᐦᒋ ᐄᔑᓈᑯᐦᒡ ᒥᔥᑏᐦ ᒑᐧᑳᓐ᙮ ᐋᑯᑎᐦ ᑳ ᐅᐦᒋ ᒫᒥᑐᓈᔪᐦᑎᒥᐦᐄᑯᑦ ᐧᒑᓂᓀᓐ ᐋᑯᔥ ᐋᑳ ᒑ ᐧᐄᐦ ᑮᑲᑖᑦ ᐊᓂᔫ ᐋᐦ ᔖᑳᐅᐱᔪᑦ᙮

ᐋᑳ ᑖᐧᐸᐅᒑᔪᒦᓯᑦ, ᐋᐦ ᓈᓂᑭᓯᒌᑦ, ᐧᒑᓂᓀᓐ ᑳ ᐧᐄᐦᑎᒧᐧᐋᑦ ᐹᔪᒄ ᐊᓂᔫᐦ ᐅᐧᐄᒑᐧᐋᑭᓐᐦ ᐋᐦ ᔖᑳᐅᐱᔪᑦ᙮ ᐧᐋᐦ, ᐄᑎᑯ = ᑭᔫᐦ ᒧᔫᒻ ᐋᑳ ᐃᔫᐱᑖᔪᒥᑯᑦ ᑳᐦ ᐃᐦᑐᑖᑯᑦ, ᒧᔫᒻ ᐊᓂᑖᐦ ᒑ ᑳᐦᒋᔥᑎᓂᒥᔪᒡᐦ ᐊᓂᔫ ᐅᑖᐦᑯᓯᐧᐃᓐ ᐋᐦ ᐄᐦᑎᔪᒡᐦ᙮ ᒋᔅᒑᔪᐦᑖᑯᓐ ᐱᔥᒡ ᒑᐧᑳᓐ ᐋᑳ ᓂᐦᑖ ᐄᔪᐦᒡ ᒑ ᒌᐦ ᐄᔑᓈᑯᐦᒡ ᐱᑯᓂᒑ ᐊᓐ ᐋᐦ ᒫᔫᔪᒫᑭᓂᐧᐃᑦ ᐊᐧᐋᓐ ᐊᓂᑖᐦ ᒫᐧᑳᒡ ᐋᐦ ᐄᐦᑖᑦ ᑳ ᐄᔥᐹᔪᒡ ᒋᔅᑯᑎᒫᑰᑭᒥᑯᐦᒡ᙮ ᐋᑯᑎᐦ ᑳ ᐄᑖᔪᐦᑎᐦᒃ ᐧᒑᓂᓀᓐ ᐋᑳ ᐋᑯᔥ ᒑ ᒋᔅᒑᔪᐦᑎᔪᐧᐋᑦ ᐋᐦ ᔖᑳᐅᐱᔪᑦ᙮

ᐅᔫ ᒫᒃ ᐹᐳᓂᔪᒡ ᐧᒑᓂᓀᓐ ᑳ ᑯᐧᑖᔖᐳᐳᐧᓈᓯᑦ, ᑳ ᓂᐱᐦᐋᑦ ᒋᔖᔫᒄᐦ, ᓃᔥᑎᓂᐅᓈᐤ ᒥᓯᑦ ᒌᐦ ᐄᔅᐱᓯᓈᑯᓯᔪᐤᐦ, ᐊᔑᐧᑳᐱᐦᒋᑭᓂᔪᐤ ᐋᐦ ᐋᐱᒋᔥᑖᑦ᙮ ᐊᓂᔫ ᑳ ᐄᔑ ᒋᔅᑯᑎᒫᒑᔪᒡᐦ ᒋᔖᔪᔪᐤᐦ ᔫᔪᑖ ᓈᐦᐋᐤ ᐋᐦ ᑭᓂᐧᐋᐱᒥᑐᒡ ᐊᓂᔫᐦ ᒋᔖᔫᒄᐦ ᐋᑯᑖᐦ ᑳ ᐃᐦᑎᒃ ᐋᐦᐧᒫᔫᐦ ᐹᔅᒋᐧᔖᑦ᙮ ᐊᓂᔫ ᒫᒃ ᑳ ᔖᑳᐅᐱᔪᑦ ᐋᔥᒄ ᓂᒥ ᐊᐧᐋᔪᐤᐦ ᐅᐦᒋ ᒋᔅᒑᔪᐦᑎᔫᐤ᙮

ᒫᒃ ᑲᔦ ᐊᓂᔮ ᐧᐁᑖᒡ ᐁ ᒪᔅᑲᐧᐃᔪᑦ ᒨᔥ ᐁ ᓴᓵᐅᐸᔪᐦᐅᑦ᙮ ᑏᐧᐁᐦᒡ ᒌ ᓂᔥᑰᔥᑕᐧᐁᐤ ᓰᐦᒃ ᑳ ᐅᑖᒪᐦᐧᐋᑦ ᓇᐦᐋᐤ ᐅᔅᑲᐦᑎᑯᔪᒡ᙮ ᑳ ᐅᑎᔑᐸᔪᐦᐅᔪᒡ ᐊᓂᔮ ᓈᐯᓴ ᑲ ᐊᑎ ᐸᐦᒋᔑᓂᔪᒡ᙮ ᐧᐁᐃᐱᔅᒌᔥ ᐁᐅᒄ ᑳ ᐃᔑᓂᔪᒡ ᐁ ᐁᑎᒋᓂᔑᓂᔪᒡ, ᑫᒃ ᑳ ᐧᐊᓂᔥᑳᑦ, ᓇᒧᐃ ᒫᒃ ᒦᓐ ᓂᐦᑖ ᐅᐦᒋ ᐱᔅᑫᔪᒥᑰ ᐊᓂᔮ ᓇᐯᓴ᙮ ᓇᒧᐃ ᓈᔅᒡ ᒋᓄᐅᔥ ᐅᔮ ᑳ ᐃᔅᐸᔪᑦ ᐧᒑᓇᓀᓐ ᐊᓂᑕ ᒋᔅᑯᑕᒫᑫᐅᑲᒥᑯᐦᒡ ᒌ ᐊᔪᒥᑐᑖᑲᓅ ᐁ ᓇᓈᑕᐦᑯᐦᐄᑐᓈᓅᐦᒡ᙮ ᐁᑯᑦ ᐋᐦᒌᐤ ᑳ ᐊᑎ ᐃᔅᐸᔪᐦᒡ᙮ ᐁᒄ ᑳ ᑲᐧᑫᑌᔪᐦᑕᐦᒃ ᐧᒑᓇᓀᓐ ᑫᒌ ᐧᐄᐦᑕᐦᒃ ᐊᓂᔮ ᒨᔥ ᐁᒌ ᑳᑖᑦ᙮

ᓃᔥᑕᒻ, ᒌ ᑯᐃᑐᐧᐁᔪᐦᑕᒻ ᑫᒌ ᐧᐄᐦᑕᐦᒃ ᐁᒄ ᐯᔪᒄ ᐅᐧᐄᑫᐧᐋᑲᓐ ᑳ ᐧᐄᐦᑕᒧᐧᐋᑦ ᐁ ᓰᐧᐋᑲᒥᐦᐧᑫᑦ᙮ "ᑖᐧᐯ ᐋ," ᒌ ᐃᐧᑌᔮ ᐁᒄ ᓇᒧᐃ ᒦᓐ ᐅᐦᒋ ᐋᐸᑌᔪᒥᑰ, ᐧᑫᒡ ᑮᐹ ᐁ ᒫᔫᑕᓂᔪᒡ ᐁ ᓰᐧᐋᑲᒥᐦᐧᑫᑦ᙮ ᐁᐅᒄ ᑮᐹ ᐯᔪᒄ ᑫᐧᑳᓐ ᓇᒧᐃ ᐧᐄᔅᑳᑦ ᒋᑲᒌ ᐋᐦᑎᓂᑲᓅ ᐊᓂᑌ ᒋᔅᑯᑕᒫᑫᐅᑲᒥᑯᐦᒡ ᐁᐅᑰ ᑫᒌ ᒫᔦᔪᒥᑯᔪᓐ ᒥᒄ ᐊᓐ ᐅᐦᒋ ᐋᐦᒌᐤ ᐁ ᐃᔑᓈᑯᓯᔪᓐ ᒫᒃ ᐁ ᐃᑌᔪᐦᑖᑯᓯᔪᓐ᙮ ᐁᐅᒄ ᒫᒃ ᐅᔮ ᐧᐁᐦᒋ ᐃᑌᔪᐦᑕᐦᒃ ᐧᒑᓇᓀᓐ ᐁᑯᔥ ᐁᑳ ᑫ ᐅᐦᒋ ᐧᐄᐦᑕᒧᐧᐋᑦ ᑯᑕᒃ ᐊᐧᐁᔮᐦ ᐁ ᓰᐧᐋᑲᒥᐦᐧᑫᑦ᙮

ᐊᓂᔮ ᐯᐳᓂᔪᒡ ᑳ ᑯᐧᑖᓵᐳᓄᓯᑦ ᐧᒑᓇᓀᓐ, ᑳᑰᔥ ᒌ ᓂᐸᐦᐁᐤ᙮ ᓃᔥᑐᓅᓄᐤ ᒥᓯᑦ ᒌ ᐃᔅᐱᔑᓈᑯᓯᔮ ᑳ ᐹᔅᒋᐧᓵᑦ 7 ᑳ ᐃᒋᔥᑌᔪᒡ ᐹᔅᒋᔑᑲᓐ ᔑᐧᑳᐱᐦᒋᑲᓂᔮ ᐁᒌ ᐋᐸᒋᐦᑖᑦ᙮ ᒌ ᓇᓈᑲᑐᐧᐁᔪᐦᑕᒻ ᒋᒉᐃᓅ ᐅᒋᔅᑯᑕᒫᑫᐧᐃᓂᔮ, ᐹᑎᔥ ᑫᓇᐧᐋᐸᒥᑯᑦ ᐊᓂᔮᐦ ᑳᑰᔥ ᐁᒄ ᔫᒄ ᑳ ᐹᔅᒋᐧᓵᑦ᙮ ᐁᔅᒄ ᑮᐹ ᓇᒧᐃ ᐊᐧᐁᔮᐦ ᐅᐦᒋ ᒋᔅᑫᔪᒥᑰ ᑖᓐ ᐁ ᐄᑖᔅᐱᓄᑦ᙮

l'avaient rendu plus fort. Il se releva et lui asséna un solide coup de poing sur le front. Le gars encaissa le coup et tomba au sol. Il demeura allongé sur le dos pendant un moment, puis se releva et n'embêta plus jamais Jonathan. Peu de temps après, l'école mit en place un programme anti-intimidation. Les choses commençaient à changer. Jonathan commença à penser à dévoiler son secret.

made him. He just wound up and landed one solid punch to the forehead. The guy buckled and hit the ground. He lay there on his back for a while, then got up and never bothered Jonathan again. Soon after that, the school brought in an anti-bullying program. Things were beginning to change. Jonathan began to think about letting his secret out.

En guise d'essai, avec hésitation, Jonathan mentionna à l'un de ses amis qu'il était diabétique. « Ah », dit son ami – et il commença à éviter Jonathan comme si celui-ci avait une maladie contagieuse au lieu du diabète. Certaines choses, comme le fait d'être mal traité à l'école secondaire si on était différent, ne changeraient probablement jamais. Pour Jonathan, la voie du secret demeurait celle à suivre.

Tentatively, hesitantly, Jonathan mentioned to one of his friends that he had diabetes. "Huh," his friend said – and began avoiding him, as if he had something contagious instead of diabetes. Some things, like being treated badly in high school if you were different, would probably never change. For Jonathan, secrecy was still the way to go.

L'année où Jonathan eut 16 ans, il tua un ours. À 24 pieds de distance, 7 mm avec une lunette. Comme les aînés le lui avait enseigné, il prit soin d'établir un contact visuel complet avec l'ours avant de tirer. Son diabète était toujours un secret.

The year Jonathan turned 16, he killed a bear. 24 feet away, 7mm with a scope. Like the Elders taught, he was careful to make full eye contact with the bear before shooting. The diabetes was still a secret.

ᐊᓂᔮ ᒫᒃ ᓃᐧᓵᓵᑉ ᑳ ᐃᐦᑎᐦᑐᐳᐧᓈᓯᑦ ᐧᒑᓂᑲᓐ, ᐋᑯᑎᐦ ᑳᐦ ᓂᑎᐧᐋᔨᒥᑯᑦ ᒨᓂᔨᐠ ᐁᐃ ᒑ ᐧᐄᒋᐦᐋᑦ ᒑ ᓈᑎᒧᐧᐋᑦ ᑭᔨᐧᐹ᙮ ᓂᒥ ᐅᐦᒋ ᒥᔪᐱᔨᔨᐤ ᒑᐧᑳᔨᐤ ᒑ ᒌᐦ ᒫᑎᐧᐋᑦ ᐊᓂᑎᐦ, ᐋᑯᐦ ᒦᓐ ᒦᔥᑯᒡ ᐊᑎ ᐱᐳᓂᔨᒑ ᒑ ᑯᒋᐦᑖᑦ, ᒥᒄ ᒫᒃ ᐋᔭᐱᔅ ᒌᐦ ᒥᐧᔮᔨᐦᑎᒻ ᐋᐦ ᒌᐦ ᑯᐧᑳᒋᒥᑯᑦ᙮ ᐊᓂᔮ ᒫᒃ ᐹᐳᓂᔨᒡ ᒦᓐ ᒌᐦ ᒋᒋᔥᑖᐤ ᐋᐦ ᐋᐱᒋᐦᑖᑦ ᐄᓐᓯᓇᓐ᙮ ᐋᔭᐱᔅ ᒫᒃ ᐋᔥᒄ ᓂᒥ ᐅᐦᒋ ᐧᐄᐦᑎᒧᐧᐋᐤ ᐊᐧᐋᔨᐤᐦ ᐋᐦ ᓵᑳᐅᐱᔨᑦ᙮

ᐊᓂᑎᐦ ᒫᒃ ᐊᓂᔮ ᒫᐧᑳᒡ ᑳ ᐄᔅᐱᔨᔨᒡ, ᐊᓂᒌ ᐄᔨᔨᐤ ᓂᑐᐦᑯᔨᓂᔨᐤ ᑳᓂᐧᐋᐱᐦᑎᐦᒡ (ᐋᐦ ᒌᐦ ᑭᓂᐧᐋᔨᐦᑎᐦᒡᐦ ᐋᔅᐱᔨᐦᐄᐧᐋᔨᒡ ᐋᐦ ᓵᑳᐅᐱᔨᓈᓂᐧᐃᐧᐃᔨᒡ) ᒌᐦ ᑯᐧᑳᒋᒫᐧᐃᒡ ᐧᒑᓂᑲᓐᐦ ᒑ ᒌᐦ ᐧᐄᒋᐦᐄᑯᒡ, ᒑ ᒌᐦ ᐋᔨᒧᑎᒥᔨᒡᐦ ᐊᓂᔮ ᐋᐦ ᓵᑳᐅᐱᔨᓈᓂᐧᐃᐧᐃᔨᒡ ᐋᔅᐱᐦᐄᑯᑦ ᐧᐄᔨ ᐧᒑᓂᑲᓐ, ᒑ ᐋᔨᒥᐦᐋᑦ ᐊᓂᔮᐦ ᐋᐱᑎᓰᓰᐦ ᑭᔮᐦ ᓂᑐᐦᑯᔨᓂᔅᐧᑳᐤᐦ᙮ ᒌᐦ ᓂᔅᑯᒨ ᒫᒃ, ᒥᒄ ᐋᑳ ᑭᔨᐧᐹ ᑯᑎᒃᐦ ᐊᐧᐋᔨᐤᐦ ᒋᔅᒑᔨᐦᑎᔮᑭᓂᐧᐄᒋᐦᐋ ᐊᓂᔮ ᐋᐦ ᐄᑖᔅᐱᓈᑦ᙮ ᐋᔑᒄ ᒫᒃ ᐊᓂᔮ ᐋᔨᒥᐦᐋᒡᐦ ᐊᓂᔮᐦ ᐋᐱᑎᓰᓰᐦ, ᑭᔮᐦ ᒥᓯᐧᐋ ᒌᐦ ᐧᐄᐦᑎᒧᐧᐋᐤ ᐊᓂᔮ ᐋᑎ ᐃᔨᑖᔨᐦᑎᒥᐦᐄᑯᑦ ᒫᐧᑳᔨᐤ ᑭᔮᐦ ᑖᓐ ᒥᒄ ᐊᓂᔮ ᐋᔑ ᒋᔅᒑᔨᐦᑎᐦᒃ = ᒥᒄ ᒫᒃ ᒥᓯᐧᐋ ᒌᐦ ᐧᐄᐦᑎᒧᐧᐋᐤ ᐊᓂᔮᐦ ᑳ ᐋᔨᒥᐦᐋᑦ ᐋᑳ ᓈᔥᑎᔨᒡ ᒑ ᐧᐄᐦᑎᒥᔨᒡᐦ ᐧᐄᔨ ᐊᓂᔮ ᐋᐦ ᓵᑳᐅᐱᔨᑦ᙮ ᑖᐹ ᐧᐋᐦᑎᓐ ᐆ ᐋᐦ ᐄᔑᑳᑖᑭᓂᐧᐃᒡ ᒫᐧᑳᓐ᙮

ᐊᓂᔮ ᒫᒃ ᓈᐧᐋᐤ ᑳ ᒌᔑ ᐋᔨᒥᑦ, ᑳᐦ ᐄᑐᐦᑖᑦ ᐊᓂᑖᐦ ᒑ ᑯᐧᑳᒋᐦᐄᓯᑦ ᐋᐦ ᐧᐋᐧᐋᐹᔅᑯᐦᐄᒐᓂᐧᐃᐧᐃᔨᒡ᙮ ᐹᑎᒫᐦ ᒫᒃ, ᒫᐧᑳᒡ ᐋᐦ ᐱᒧᐦᑖᑦ ᐋᐦ ᒌᐧᐋᑦ, ᐊᓂᑖᐦ ᐋᐦ ᐱᒧᐦᑖᓂᐧᐃᐧᐃᔨᒡ ᐋᔑ ᐱᒋᔅᑎᓂᐦᒃ ᐊᓂᔮ

ᑳ ᓃᐧᓵᓵᐳᓄᓯᑦ ᒫᒃ, ᓈᔅᒡ ᒌ ᑳᔅᒋᐦᐆ ᐦᐊᑮ ᐁ ᒉᑐᐧᐁᑦ ᐁᒄ ᑳ ᐧᐄᓵᒫᑲᓅᑦ ᒉᒌ ᐧᐄᒋᐦᐋᑦ ᑳ ᐋᐦᐧᑳᑎᓰᐧᑖᐤ᙮ ᓇᒧᐃ ᐅᐦᒋ ᒥᔫᐸᔫ ᐅᔫ ᑳᐧᐄ ᐃᐦᑎᑦ ᒥᒄ ᑮᐹ ᒌ ᒥᔮᑲᓅ ᐁᔅᒄ ᒦᓐ ᒉᒌ ᑯᒋᐦᑖᑦ ᐊᓂᔫ ᒦᓐ ᐱᐳᓂᔨᒉ, ᒋᐦᒋᐧᐁ ᒫᒃ ᒌ ᑌᔨᐦᑕᒥᐦᐄᑰ ᐁᒌ ᑲᐧᑫᒋᒫᑲᓅᑦ ᒉᒌ ᐧᐄᒋᒉᑐᐧᐁᒫᑦ ᐊᓂᔫᐦ᙮ ᐊᓂᔫ ᒫᒃ ᑳ ᐱᐳᓂᔨᒡ ᐁᑯᑦ ᑳ ᒋᐦᒋᐸᔨᔨᒡ ᐁ ᐸᒋᔅᑲᐦᐆᓯᑦ᙮ ᔮᐸᒡ ᒫᒃ ᒌ ᑳᑖᐤ ᐊᓂᔫ ᐁ ᓰᐧᐋᑲᒥᐦᐧᑫᑦ᙮

ᐁᑯᑦ ᒫᒃ ᐊᓂᑕ ᐧᐃᔭᔅ ᐊᓂᑌ ᐅᐦᒋ ᒥᔫᐱᒫᑎᓰᐧᐃᓐ ᐁ ᓇᓈᒋᐦᑖᑲᓅᐦᒡ (ᐊᓂᑌ ᑫᓇᐧᐁᔨᐦᑖᑲᓄᔨᐧᑳᐤ ᐅᒪᓯᓇᐦᐄᑲᓐᐦ ᐁ ᓰᐧᐋᑲᒥᐦᐧᑫᑦ) ᒌ ᑲᐧᑫᒋᒫᑲᓅ ᒉᒌ ᑎᐹᒋᒥᓯᑦ ᐁ ᓰᐧᐋᑲᒥᐦᐧᑫᑦ ᐊᓂᑌ ᐁ ᓂᔥᑐᐧᐄᔨᒡ ᓂᑐᐦᑯᐃᓂᔅᐧᑫᐤ ᑳ ᐧᐄᒑᐸᑎᓰᒪᔨᒡ ᑲᔭ ᓂᑐᐦᑯᐃᓂᔅᐧᑫᐤᐦ᙮ ᒌ ᑖᐧᐯᐦᑕᒻ ᐅᔫ ᑳ ᐃᔑ ᑲᐧᑫᒋᒫᑲᓅᑦ ᒥᒄ ᒌ ᐃᐧᑌᐤ ᐁᑳ ᒉᒌ ᐧᐄᐦᑕᒧᐧᐋᔨᒡ ᑯᑕᒃ ᐊᐧᐁᔫ᙮ ᑕᐦᐧᑖᐤ ᑳ ᑎᐹᒋᒥᓯᑦ ᐊᓂᑕ ᐁ ᒫᒨᐱᔨᐧᑖᐤ ᓂᑐᐦᑯᐃᓐ ᐋᐸᑎᓰᓰᐦ, ᒌ ᐧᐄᐦᑕᒧᐧᐁᐤ ᑖᓐ ᑳᐯᒋ ᐃᔅᐸᔨᑦ ᐁ ᓰᐧᐋᑲᒥᐦᐧᑫᑦ ᐁ ᐧᐄᐦᑕᒧᐧᐋᑦ ᑖᓐ ᑖᓐ ᐁ ᐃᔑ ᒋᔅᒉᔨᐦᑕᐦᒃ ᒉᒌ ᐅᐦᒋ ᒋᔅᒉᔨᐦᑕᒦᐧᑖᐤ ᐊᓂᔫ ᑳ ᐋᔨᒥᐦᐋᑦ ᐊᐧᐁᔫᐦ = ᒥᒄ ᔮᐸᒡ ᐁᑯᓐ ᒨᔥ ᑳᒌ ᐄᑖᑦ ᐁᑳ ᒉᒌ ᐧᐄᐦᑕᒧᐧᐋᔨᒡ ᐊᐧᐁᔫᐦ ᐁ ᓰᐧᐋᑲᒥᐦᐧᑫᑦ᙮ ᑖᐧᐯ ᒌ ᐋᐸᑎᓰᐦᑲᐦᑕᒻ ᐁᐧᐄ ᑳᑖᑦ ᐅᔫ᙮

ᐃᔅᑯᑕᒃ ᓄᐧᐋᐤ ᑳ ᐊᔨᒥᑦ ᐊᓂᑌ ᐁ ᓂᔥᑐᐧᐄᓈᓄᔨᒡ, ᑳ ᒌᔑᐦᑖᑦ ᒫᒃ ᐦᐋᑮ ᒌ ᓂᑑ ᒉᑐᐧᐁᐤ ᒥᒄ ᐁ ᔅᓵᐅᐸᔨᐦᐆᓈᓄᔨᒡ᙮ ᐊᒧᐃ ᒫᒃ ᒥᐦᒉᑐ ᑎᐸᐦᐄᑲᓐᐦ ᒉᐧᑳᒡ ᐁ ᐱᒧᐦᑌᑦ ᐁ ᒌᐧᐁᑦ, ᒌ ᐸᒋᔥᑎᓇᒻ ᐧᐄᐧᐊᑦ ᐊᓂᑕ ᐹᐦᒋᔥᑎᓂᔨᐧᑳᐤ

L'année où Jonathan eut 17 ans, une équipe de hockey junior AAA voulut qu'il devienne leur homme fort. Cela ne fonctionna pas, et il pourrait essayer de nouveau l'année suivante, mais cela faisait un petit velours de se le voir proposer. Cette année-là, il dut également recommencer à prendre de l'insuline. Et son diabète était toujours un secret.

Vers cette époque, le Conseil cri de la santé (qui tenait un dossier sur son diabète) demanda à Jonathan de faire des présentations sur son diabète aux représentants de la santé communautaire et aux infirmières. Il accepta, mais seulement si aucune personne à l'extérieur de la salle ne le découvrait. Lors de chaque présentation, devant une salle remplie de travailleurs de la santé, il décrivait son expérience et donnait tous les renseignements et les aperçus possibles, mais il demandait que chaque personne dans la salle garde son état confidentiel. Garder un secret demandait tellement de travail.

Après la quatrième présentation, il alla à son entraînement de hockey. Quelques heures plus tard, sur le chemin du retour, il laissa tomber son lourd sac d'équipement sur le trottoir, sortit

The year Jonathan turned 17, a Junior AAA hockey team wanted him to be their enforcer. It didn't work out, and he could try again next year, but it was nice to be asked. That year, he had to start taking insulin again too. And the diabetes was still a secret.

Around that time, the Cree Board of Health (which had record of his diabetes) asked Jonathan to give some presentations about his diabetes to Community Health Representatives and nurses. He agreed, but only if no one outside the room would find out. In every presentation, to every roomful of healthcare workers, he described his experiences and gave all the insight and information that he could – but asked that each person in the room keep his condition confidential. Secrecy was so much work.

After the fourth presentation, he went to hockey practice. A few hours later, on the way home, he dropped his heavy equipment bag on the sidewalk, pulled out his cellphone, and posted on Facebook

ᑳ ᑯᓯᑯᓂᔨᒡ ᐅᐧᐄᐦᐧᑳᔮᒻ, ᐧᑳᔨᑯᓂᐦᒃ ᐊᓂᔮ ᑳᐱᐹᑎᐦᑯᓂᑭᓂᐧᐃᔑᔨᒡ ᐋᐦ ᐋᐦᔨᒥᓈᓂᐧᐃᐧᐃᔨᒡ, ᑮᔮᐦ ᒫᓯᓈᐦᒃ ᐊᓂᑎᐦ ᒥᓯᐧᐋ ᐊᐧᐋᔨᐤᐦ ᒑ ᒌᐦ ᐧᐋᐱᐦᑎᒥᔨᒡᐦ, ᐋᐦ ᔖᑳᐅᐱᔨᑦ.

ᐋᑯᑖᐦ ᒫᒃ ᒑ ᐄᔑᓈᑯᓂᔨᒡ, ᓂᒧᐃ ᒋᑭ ᒌᐦ ᒌᐧᐋᑳᐴ. ᔕᔥ ᒫᒃ ᒥᓯᐧᐋ ᐊᐧᐋᔨᐤᐦ ᒋᑭ ᒋᔅᒑᔨᐦᑎᒥᔨᐤᐦ.

ᐊᓂᔮᐦ ᒫᒃ ᑳ ᐧᐄᒋᒫᑎᐧᐋᒪᑦ ᐋᐦ ᐧᐋᐧᐋᐹᔅᑯᓐᐦᐄᒑᓂᐧᐃᐧᐃᔨᒡ, ᓂᒧᐃ ᓈᔥᑎᔨᒡ ᐅᐦᒋ ᐃᔮᐱᒑᔨᐦᑎᒥᔨᐤᐦ. ᐋᔥᒄ ᐧᐄ ᐋᐦ ᓈᑎᒧᐧᐋᑦ ᐅᐧᐄᒪᐧᑳᑭᓐᐦ, ᒑ ᒌᐦ ᒧᔥᑖᐦᒋᐦᐧᐋᑦ ᐊᓂᔮᐦ ᐧᑳᒋᐦᐋᒡ, ᓂᒧᐃ ᐧᐄᔮᔥ ᐄᔑᓈᑯᓂᔮᐤ ᐋᑦ ᐊᓂᔮ ᐋᐦ ᔖᑳᐅᐱᔨᑦ. ᐊᓂᔮᐦ ᐅᒋᔥᐧᑳᔑᔒᒻᐦ ᐊᓂᔮᐦ ᑳ ᑳᑐᐧᐋᑦ ᑮᔮᐦ, ᓂᒧᐃ ᐅᐦᒋ ᐃᔮᐱᒑᔨᐦᑎᒥᔨᐤᐦ. ᑖᓐ ᒑ ᐃᔨᓃᒡ ᐧᐋᔥ ᓈᔥᑖᐧᐹᐦ ᒥᒥᔫᐦᑭᐧᐋᐤ ᑮᔮᐦ ᑯᐃᔅᒄ ᐃᐦᑐᑎᐧᐋᐤ.

ᐊᓂᔮ ᒫᐅᒡ ᑳ ᑯᔥᑯᐦᐄᑯᑦ ᐋᔪᐧᐃᒄ ᐊᓂᔮ ᑳ ᐄᔑ ᓂᔥᐧᑳᐅᔑᐦᑖᔨᒡᐦ ᐹᔨᒄ ᐊᓂᔮᐦ ᑳ ᒋᔅᑯᑎᒫᒑᔨᒡᐦ ᐊᓂᑖᐦ ᑳ ᐄᔥᐹᔨᒡ ᒋᔅᑯᑎᒫᑑᑭᒥᑯᐦᒡ ᐋᐦ ᒌᐦ ᔖᑳᐅᐱᔨᔨᒡᐦ ᑮᔮᐦ: "ᒋᒋᔅᒑᔨᐦᑖᓐ ᐋ," ᐄᑎᑯ ᐊᓂᔮᐦ ᒋᔅᑯᑎᒫᒑᓰᐦ ᐹᔨᐧᑳᐤ ᐋᐦ ᒌᔑᑳᔨᒡ, "ᒌᔮᓂᐤ ᐋᐦ ᔖᑳᐅᐱᔨᔨᒄ, ᑖᐹ ᐊᑐᒡ ᒋᒫᑎᐧᐋᓈᓂᐤ ᐋᐦ ᐧᐋᐧᐋᐹᔅᑯᐦᐄᒑᓂᐧᐃᒡ. ᐧᐋᔅ ᓂᒥ ᒫᒥᓈᑎᓰᓈᓂᐆ."

ᓰᐦᒃ ᒌᐦ ᑯᒋᔥᑖᐤ ᐧᒐᓂᓀᓐ ᐋᑳ ᒑ ᒌᐦ ᐹᐦᐱᑦ. ᓂᒧᐃ ᐅᐦᒋ ᐧᐄᐦ ᒫᔮᔨᐦᒋᒑᐤ ᒥᒄ ᒫᒃ ᔕᔥ ᓃᓱᐱᐳᓐᐦ ᓂᒥ ᐅᐦᒋ ᐋᐱᒋᐦᒑᐤ ᓂᑑᐦᑯᔨᓂᔨᐤ

ᐅᒣᑐᐧᐁᐅᒉᐧᑳᓂᒻᐦ ᐅᑖᐦᑳᐱᐦᒉᓂᑲᓂᔥ ᑳ ᑯᐃᑯᓇᐦᒃ ᐅᐧᐹᑲᑎᒥᐦᒡ, ᐁᒄ ᑳ ᒪᓯᓇᐦᐄᒉᑦ ᐊᓂᑕ ᕓᐃᔅᐳᒃ ᐁ ᐧᐄᐦᑕᐦᒃ ᐧᐄᔭ ᐧᒑᓇᓀᓐ ᓚᓐᑕᓐ ᐁ ᐊᔮᑦ ᑳᓰᐧᐋᑲᒥᐦᐧᑳᓄᔨᒡ.

ᐁᑯᑦ ᒫᒃ, ᓵᔅ ᒌ ᐧᐄᐦᑕᒻ. ᓵᔅ ᒥᓯᐧᐁ ᐊᐧᐁᓐ ᒋᔅᒉᔨᐦᑕᒻ.

ᐊᓂᔫᐦ ᐦᐋᑮ ᑳ ᐧᐄᒋᒣᑐᐧᐁᒫᑦ ᓇᒧᐃ ᐧᐃᓭᔅ ᐅᐦᒋ ᐃᑌᔨᐦᑕᒥᐦᐄᑯᔫᐦ ᐁ ᓰᐧᐋᑲᒥᐦᐧᑫᑦ. ᑌᐱᔮᐦᒡ ᐁ ᐋᐦᐧᑳᑎᓰᑦ ᐁ ᑯᑎᔅᑯᐧᐋᑦ ᐊᓂᔫᐦ ᑳ ᑭᒋᐦᐧᐋᐧᑖᐤ ᐁ ᑯᔥᑎᑯᑦ ᒫᒃ ᐁᐅᒄ ᒥᒄ ᐊᓂᔫ ᑳ ᑲᓇᐧᐋᐸᐦᑕᒥᔨᒡ. ᐅᒋᔅᐧᑫᓰᒻ ᑲᓭ ᓵᔅ ᐧᐁᔅᑲᒡ ᒌ ᒋᔅᒉᔨᐦᑕᒥᔫ ᐁ ᓰᐧᐋᑲᒥᐦᐧᑫᔨᒡ ᐧᒑᓇᓀᓐ ᒥᒄ ᓇᒧᐃ ᐧᐄᔅᑲᒡ ᐅᐦᒋ ᐧᐄᐦᑕᒧᐧᐁᐤ ᐊᐧᐁᔫᐦ. ᒌ ᒥᔫᐦᑲᑰ ᐁᒄ ᓇᒧᐃ ᐅᐦᒋ ᐸᐹᒣᔨᐦᑕᒥᐦᐄᑰ ᐁ ᓰᐧᐋᑲᒥᐦᐧᑫᔨᒡ.

ᐊᓂᔫ ᐯᔭᒄ ᒉᐧᑳᔫ ᑳ ᑯᔥᐧᑫᔨᐦᑕᒥᐦᐄᑯᑦ ᐧᒑᓇᓀᓐ ᐊᓂᑌ ᒋᔅᑯᑕᒫᒉᐅᑲᒥᑯᐦᒡ ᒌ ᐃᐦᑖᔫ ᐯᔭᒄ ᓈᐯᐤ ᒋᔅᑯᑕᒫᒉᓰᐦ ᐁ ᓰᐧᐋᑲᒥᐦᐧᑫᔨᒡ. ᐯᔭᐧᑳᐤ ᒌ ᐄᑎᑰ, "ᒋ ᒋᔅᒉᔨᐦᑌᓐ ᐋ ᒉᐧᑳᓐ. ᒋᔮᓅ ᑳ ᓰᐧᐋᑲᒥᐦᐧᑫᔨᐦᒄ ᓇᒧᐃ ᒋᐹ ᐅᐦᒋ ᒣᑕᐧᐁᓈᓅ ᐦᐋᑮ. ᐧᐁᓰ ᑯᔥᑖᑎᑯᓐ."

ᓇᒧᐃ ᐅᐦᒌ ᐃᐦᑑ ᐧᒑᓇᓀᓐ ᐁᑳ ᒉᒌ ᐹᐦᐱᑦ ᐊᓂᔫ ᑳ ᐃᐧᑌᔨᒡ. ᓇᒧᐃ ᑮᐹ ᐧᐄ ᐁ ᒫᓭᔨᒫᑦ ᒥᒄ ᒌ ᐃᐦᑑ ᓃᓱ ᐱᐳᓐᐦ ᐁᑳ ᐅᐦᒋ ᐅᑎᓇᐦᒃ

son téléphone cellulaire et afficha sur Facebook que lui, Jonathan Linton, était diabétique.

that he, Jonathan Linton, had diabetes.

Il n'y avait pas de retour en arrière possible. Désormais, tout le monde était au courant.

There was no going back. Now, everyone knew.

Il s'avéra que cela importait peu à son équipe de hockey. S'il demeurait le meilleur homme fort du coin, s'il continuait à inspirer la peur dans les cœurs de l'équipe adverse, cela n'avait pas d'importance. Cela importait également peu à sa petite amie, qui était au courant depuis un certain temps, mais gardait le secret. S'il la traitait bien, quelle importance ?

His hockey team, it turned out, didn't actually care. If he was still the best enforcer around, if he still struck fear into the opposing team, it didn't matter. His girlfriend, who had known for a while but kept the secret, also didn't care. If he treated her well, what did it matter?

Le plus surprenant, fut la réaction d'un enseignant du secondaire qui était lui-même diabétique : « Tu sais, dit un jour le professeur. Nous, les diabétiques, ne devrions pas jouer au hockey. C'est trop brutal ».

What was more surprising was the response of a high school teacher who himself had diabetes: "You know," the teacher said one day, "We diabetics shouldn't play hockey. It's too rough."

Jonathan prit sur lui pour ne pas rire. Il ne voulait pas être grossier, mais il avait passé deux ans sans avoir besoin

It was all Jonathan could do not to laugh. He didn't mean to be rude but he had gone for two years without medication or

ᑮᔮᐦ ᐄᓐᓯᓕᓐ ᐋᔫᐧᐃᒄ ᐋᑯᐦ ᐊᓂᔮᐦ ᒨᔥ
ᐋᐦ ᒌᐦ ᔖᔖᐧᐋᑦ᙮ ᓈᔥᒡ ᐋᐦ ᒌᐦ ᐧᐄᒋᐦᐄᑯᑦ
ᓃᐦᑖᒡ ᒑ ᐄᔅᐱᔭᔭᒡ ᐊᓂᔮ ᐅᔖᑳᒼ ᐅᐦᒋ
ᐊᓂᔮ ᐋᐦ ᔖᔖᐧᐋᑦ᙮ ᓃᔥᑎᒼ ᐊᐧᑳᑖᔭᐦᑎᐦᒃ
ᐧᒑᓂᕋᓐ, ᑖᐹ ᓇᔥᒡ ᓂᑭ ᐃᔮᐱᑖᔮᐦᑎᐧᒫᓐ
ᐊᓂᔮ ᑳ ᐄᔑ ᐧᐄᐦᑎᐦᒃ᙮ ᐹᑎᔥ ᐹᑎᒫᐦ ᑳ
ᐄᑖᔭᐦᑎᐦᒃ ᒑᐧᑳᔭᐤ ᐊᓂᔮ ᒑ ᒋᔅᒋᓰᑎᑎᐦᒃ᙮
ᐆ ᒫ ᒋᔅᑯᑎᒫᒐᓰ ᐊᓂᑖᐦ ᑳ ᐄᔥᐹᔭᒡ ᐋᐦ
ᒋᔅᑯᑎᒫᒐᑦ, ᐋᐦ ᒌᐦ ᒋᔅᑯᑎᒫᓯᑦ ᒥᔥᑏᐦ ᐅᐦᒋ
ᐋᐦ ᔕᑳᐅᐱᔭᓈᓂᐧᐃᐧᐃᔭᒡ, ᐋᐦ ᑖᐧᐹᐦᑎᐦᒃ
ᐅᔮ ᒫᐧᑳᔭᐤ ᓈᔥᑎᔭᒡ ᐋᑳ ᑖᐧᐹᒥᑭᓂᔭᒡ, ᔖᔥ
ᓈᓂᑎᐤ ᐅᑎᒋᐱᔭᒋᒫ ᒐ ᒋᔅᒑᔭᐦᑎᔭᐧᐋᓂᐧᐃᒡ
ᒑᐧᑳᓐ ᐅᐦᒋ ᐋᐦ ᔕᑳᐅᐱᔭᓈᓂᐧᐃᒡ᙮

ᐊᓅᐦᒡ ᒫᒃ ᐅᔮ ᑳᔑᑳᔭᒡ, ᐧᒑᓂᕋᓐ ᐊᓐᑖᐦ ᐄᔑ
ᓂᑐᐦᑯᔭᓈᐱᑎᓰᐧᐃᓂᐦᒡ ᐄᔑ ᐋᐱᑎᓰᐤ ᐋᐦ
ᐧᐋᐧᐄᐦᑎᒧᐧᐋᑦ ᑮᔮᐦ ᐋᐦ ᒋᔅᑯᑎᒧᐧᐋᑦ ᐊᐧᐋᔭᐤᐦ
ᐊᑎᑎᐤ ᒑ ᒌᐦ ᒥᔫᐱᒫᑎᓯᔭᒡᐦ᙮ ᓈᔥᒡ ᐋᐦ
ᒥᐧᔫᔭᐦᑎᐦᒃ ᐊᓂᔮ ᐋᐦ ᐄᑖᐱᑎᓰᑦ᙮ ᐧᐄᒋᐦᐄᑰ
ᐋᑳ ᒐ ᐧᐃᓂᒋᔅᒋᓯᑦ ᒐ ᒌᐦ ᒥᔪᑭᓂᐧᐋᔭᒦᓯᑦ
ᑮᔮᐦ ᐋᐦ ᓂᒋᔥᑭᐧᐋᑦ ᑯᑎᒃᐦ ᐊᐧᐋᔭᐤᐦ ᑮᔮᐦ ᐋᐦ
ᐧᐋᐧᐄᒋᐦᐋᑦ᙮ ᐧᐋᐦᒌᔭᑰ ᔖᔥ ᐋᐦ ᐃᔫᔭᒧᑎᐦᒃ ᐋᐦ
ᔕᑳᐅᐱᔭᓈᓂᐧᐃᐧᐃᔭᒡ ᑮᔮᐦ ᐋᐦ ᐧᐋᐧᐄᐦᑎᒧᐧᐋᑦ
ᒥᑯ ᐊᓂᔮᐦ ᐊᐧᐋᔭᐤᐦ ᐊᑎᑎᐤ ᐋᐦ ᐧᐄᐦ
ᒋᔅᒑᔭᐦᑎᒥᔭᒡᐦ ᐅᐦᒋ ᐋᐦ ᔕᑳᐅᐱᔭᓈᓂᐧᐃᐧᐃᔭᒡ᙮
ᐅᔮ ᒫᐦᒋᒡ ᑳ ᑎᐧᐃᔥᑖᔭᒡ ᒌᐦ ᐃᔫᔭᐧᒫᐅᐦᐄᑰ
ᐋᐦ ᔕᑳᐅᐱᔭᓈᓂᐧᐃᐧᐃᔭᒡ ᐊᓂᑖᐦ ᐄᔭᔭᐤ
ᐊᔭᒧᐧᐋᔫᐲᐦᒡ ᐅᑖᐦ ᐧᒫᓐᑎᓅᐧᔫᑦ ᑳ ᐅᐦᒋ
ᐹᐦᑖᑯᓂᔭᒡ᙮ ᐊᓂᑖᐦ ᐧᐄᒋᐧᐋᐦᒡ ᐋᑯᑖᐦ
ᒑᔅᑯᑎᒫᓯᑦ ᒐ ᒌᐦ ᒌᔑᐦᑖᑦ ᐊᓂᔮ ᑳ
ᐄᔥᐹᔭᒡ ᐋᐦ ᒋᔅᑯᑎᒫᓯᓈᓂᐧᐃᐧᐃᔭᒡ᙮
ᐊᓂᔮᐦ ᐅᒋᔥᐧᑳᔑᔒᒼᐦ, ᐦᐁᕋᕐ ᐦᔫᐧᐹᐃ
ᐄᓯᓂᐦᑳᓯᔭᐤᐦ, ᒫᐧᑳᒡ ᐅᑯᔑᔑᔭᐤᐦ; ᐃᔫᔅᑭᐧᐄᐤ

ᓂᑐᐦᑯᐃᓐᐦ ᒫᒃ ᒉᒌ ᐸᒋᔅᑳᐦᐆᓯᑦ ᐱᔑᒄ
ᒥᒄ ᐁᒌ ᓴᓵᐧᐃᔭᑦ᙮ ᐊᓂᔫ ᐁᒌ ᓴᓵᐧᐃᔭᑦ ᒌ
ᓃᐦᒋᐸᓂᔫ ᐅᔕᑳᒼ᙮ ᓃᔥᑕᒼ ᒌ ᐃᑌᔭᐦᑕᒼ
ᐁ ᒫᒥᑐᓀᔭᐦᑕᐦᒃ, ᓇᒧᐃ ᓈᔅᒡ ᓂᑲ ᐅᐦᒋ
ᐸᐱᔅᑳᑖᐤ ᐆ ᓈᐯᐤ᙮ ᒉᒃ ᒫᒃ ᐯᔮᐧᑳᐤ ᓇᒧᐃ
ᓈᔅᒡ ᒋᓄᐅᔥ ᐊᓂᑌ ᐃᔑ᙮ ᐊᓂᔫᐦ ᒋᔅᑯᑕᒫᒉᓰ,
ᒋᔅᑯᑕᒫᒉᓰ ᐋᐸᑎᓯᐧᐃᓂᔫ ᑳ ᒋᔅᒉᔭᐦᑕᒥᔭᒡ,
ᒌ ᐃᐦᑕᑯᓂᔫ ᑖᓐ ᑳ ᐃᔑ ᑲᓇᐧᐋᐸᐦᑕᒥᔭᒡ
ᐁ ᓰᐧᐋᑲᒥᐦᐧᑳᑲᓄᔭᒡ ᐁᑳ ᐅᐦᒋ ᑖᐧᐯᒪᑲᓂᔭᒡ᙮
ᐁᑯᑦ ᒫᒃ ᑳ ᐅᐦᒋ ᐃᑌᔭᐦᑕᐦᒃ ᐧᒑᓇᕋᓐ ᒉᒌ
ᒋᐦᒋᐸᔭᐦᑖᑦ ᐁ ᐋᔭᒨᑕᐦᒃ ᐁ ᓰᐧᐋᑲᒥᐦᐧᑳᑲᓄᔭᒡ᙮

ᐊᓄᐦᒌᔥ ᒫᒃ ᑳ ᒌᔑᑳᒡ, ᐊᑐᔅᑲᐧᐁᐤ
ᒥᔫᐱᒫᓯᐅᓐ ᑳ ᓇᓈᑲᒋᐦᑖᔭᒡ ᐁ ᐧᐋᐧᐄᒋᐦᐋᑦ
ᐋᐦᑯᓰᐤ ᐄᓅᐦ ᐊᓂᑕ ᐅᑎᐦᑖᐧᐃᓂᐦᒡ ᑳ
ᐃᐦᑖᔭᐧᑖᐤ᙮ ᒥᔦᔭᐦᑕᒼ ᐅᔫ ᐁ ᐄᑖᐸᑎᓯᑦ᙮
ᐁᑯᑦ ᐧᐁᐦᒋ ᒋᔅᒉᔭᐦᑕᐦᒃ ᑲᔦ ᐧᐄ ᒉᒌ
ᒥᔫᑲᓇᐧᐁᔭᒥᓯᑦᑎᔫ ᐊᐧᐁᔫᐦ ᐁ ᓇᓂᑐᐧᐋᐸᒫᑦ
ᒫᓐᐦ ᐁ ᐧᐋᐧᐄᒋᐦᐋᑦ᙮ ᐧᐁᐦᑌᔭᐦᑕᒼ ᒉᒌ
ᐊᔭᒥᑐᑕᐦᒃ ᐁ ᓰᐧᐋᑲᒥᐦᐧᑳᑲᓄᔭᒡ ᒥᒄ ᐁ
ᐃᔑᓈᑯᓯᔭᒡ ᐊᐧᐁᔫ ᐊᔭᒥᐦᐁᐤ᙮ ᐅᑖᐦᒡ ᑳ
ᑑᔥᑌᔭᒡ, ᒌ ᐯᐦᑖᑯᓰ ᐊᔭᒨᔫᐲᐦᒡ᙮ ᐧᐄ ᐃᐦᑑᑕᒼ
ᐊᓂᔫ ᐁᑳ ᐅᐦᒋ ᒌᔑᐦᑖᑦ ᑳ ᒋᔅᑯᑕᒫᓯᑦ
ᐁ ᐅᔅᒋᓃᒎᑦ ᐊᓂᑌ ᐧᐄᒋᐦᒡ ᐃᐦᑑᑕᒼ ᐅᔫ᙮
ᐅᒋᔅᐧᑫᓰᒼ ᐦᐁᕋᕐ ᐦᐆᐧᐹᐃ, ᑲᓇᐧᐁᔭᒫᐅᓯᔫ;
ᐊᔦᔅᑲᐧᐃᔫ ᒉᒌ ᐅᐦᑖᐧᐄᒫᐅᑦ ᐁᔫ ᑲᔦ ᐁᑎᑑ
ᐧᐄ ᒉᑐᐧᐁᐤ ᐦᐋᑮ᙮ ᐧᐄ ᓂᑑᐦᐆ ᑲᔦ᙮ ᓵᓴ ᒌ
ᓂᐸᐦᐁᐤ ᑳᒄ, ᑳᑰᔥ, ᐊᑎᐦᒄ, ᑲᔦ ᑯᑕᒃ ᐊᐧᐁᓵᓴ
= ᒥᒄ ᐁᔅᒄ ᓇᒧᐃ ᒨᔅ᙮

de médicaments ni d'insuline à cause de son régime sportif. L'exercice avait fait baisser son taux de sucre dans le sang. Au début, Jonathan se dit : « Je n'ai pas vraiment à m'embêter avec ce type ». Le moment d'illumination lui vint un peu plus tard : si un enseignant du secondaire, un éducateur instruit qui avait beaucoup d'expérience dans le domaine du diabète, croyait quelque chose de si aberrant au sujet de la maladie, il était temps de commencer à parler du diabète.

Aujourd'hui, Jonathan travaille comme RSC pour le Conseil cri de la santé. Il adore son travail. Cela lui rappelle de prendre soin de sa propre santé et il peut rencontrer des gens et les aider. Il parle facilement du diabète désormais, à tous ceux qui veulent en entendre parler. Pas plus tard que la semaine précédente, il a donné une entrevue en cri à la radio de la CBC. Il termine ses études secondaires en parallèle par le biais de l'enseignement à domicile. Sa petite amie, Heather Hughboy, est enceinte; il se prépare à devenir père et à jouer davantage au hockey; et à chasser. Il a tué des porcs-épics, des ours, des castors, des caribous et bien plus, mais toujours pas d'orignal.

insulin because of his exercise regime. The exercise had brought his blood sugar levels down. At first, Jonathan thought, *Well, I can't really bother with this guy too much anymore*. The *Aha*! moment came a little later. If a high school teacher, an educated educator with plenty of experience in diabetes, believed something so completely false about the disease, it was time to start talking about diabetes.

Nowadays, Jonathan works as a CHR for the Cree Board of Health. He loves the work. It reminds him to take care of his own health, and he's able to meet people and help out them out. He talks about diabetes easily now, and to anyone who wants to hear about it. Just last week, he gave an interview in Cree on CBC radio. He's finishing up high school on the side through homeschooling. His girlfriend, Heather Hughboy, is pregnant; he's getting ready to be a dad and to play more hockey. And to hunt. He's killed porcupine, bear, beaver, caribou, and more – but still no moose.

ᒑ ᐅᐦᑖᐧᐄᒫᐧᐃᐨ ᑭᔮᐦ ᐊᑎᑎᐤ ᒑ ᒫᑎᐧᐋᐨ ᐋᐦ ᐧᐋᐧᐋᐹᐢᑯᐦᐄᒑᓂᐧᐃᐧᐃᔪᒡ᙮ ᑭᔮᐦ ᒑ ᓂᑐᐦᐅᐨ᙮ ᔖᔥ ᒌᐦ ᓂᐱᐦᐋᐤ ᑳᒄᐦ, ᒋᔖᔮᒄᐦ, ᐊᒥᐢᒄᐦ, ᐊᑎᐦᒄᐦ ᑭᔮᐦ ᒥᔥᑏᐦ ᓂᓈᐦᑭᐤ ᐋᐦ ᐄᔑᓈᑯᓂᔪᒡ ᒦᒋᒥᔪᐤ᙮ ᒥᒄ ᐋᔥᒄ ᓂᒥ ᐅᐦᒋ ᒌᐦ ᓂᐱᐦᐋᐤ ᒨᔅᐦ᙮

Syllabic Chart ᐄᔨᔨᐅᔥᑖᐤ

Tableau de caractères syllabiques ᐄᓅᔥᑌᐤ

ᐁ e		ᐃ i	ᐄ ii	ᐅ u	ᐆ uu	ᐊ a	ᐋ aa		ᐤ u	ᐦ h
	ᐍ we	ᐏ wi	ᐑ wii	ᐓ wu	ᐕ wuu	ᐘ wa		ᐚ waa		
ᐯ pe	ᐻ pwe	ᐱ pi	ᐲ pii	ᐳ pu	ᐴ puu	ᐸ pa	ᐹ paa	ᑇ pwaa	ᑉ p	
ᑌ te	ᑘ twe	ᑎ ti	ᑏ tii	ᑐ tu	ᑑ tuu	ᑕ ta	ᑖ taa	ᑤ twaa	ᑦ t	
ᑫ ke	ᑵ kwe	ᑭ ki	ᑮ kii	ᑯ ku	ᑰ kuu	ᑲ ka	ᑳ kaa	ᒁ kwaa	ᒃ k	ᒄ kw
ᒉ che	ᒓ chwe	ᒋ chi	ᒌ chii	ᒍ chu	ᒎ chuu	ᒐ cha	ᒑ chaa	ᒟ chwaa	ᒡ ch	
ᒣ me	ᒭ mwe	ᒥ mi	ᒦ mii	ᒧ mu	ᒨ muu	ᒪ ma	ᒫ maa	ᒹ mwaa	ᒻ m	ᒽ mw
ᓀ ne	ᓊ nwe	ᓂ ni	ᓃ nii	ᓄ nu	ᓅ nuu	ᓇ na	ᓈ naa	ᓎ nwaa	ᓐ n	
ᓓ le	ᓝ lwe	ᓕ li	ᓖ lii	ᓗ lu	ᓘ luu	ᓚ la	ᓛ laa	ᓨ lwaa	ᓪ l	
ᓭ se	ᓷ swe	ᓯ si	ᓰ sii	ᓱ su	ᓲ suu	ᓴ sa	ᓵ saa	ᔂ swaa	ᔅ s	
ᔐ she	ᔘ shwe	ᔑ shi	ᔒ shii	ᔓ shu	ᔔ shuu	ᔕ sha	ᔖ shaa	ᔤ shwaa	ᔥ sh	
ᔦ ye	ᔰ ywe	ᔨ yi	ᔩ yii	ᔪ yu	ᔫ yuu	ᔭ ya	ᔮ yaa	ᔽ ywaa	ᔾ y	
ᕃ re	ᐧᕃ rwe	ᕆ ri	ᕇ rii	ᕈ ru	ᕉ ruu	ᕋ ra	ᕌ raa	ᕎ rwaa	ᕐ r	
ᕓ ve	ᐧᕓ vwe	ᕕ vi	ᕖ vii	ᕗ vu	ᕘ vuu	ᕙ va	ᕚ vaa	ᐧᕚ vwaa	ᕝ v/f/ph	
ᕞ the	ᐧᕞ thwe	ᕠ thi	ᕡ thii	ᕢ thu	ᕣ thuu	ᕤ tha	ᕥ thaa	ᐧᕥ thwaa	ᕦ th	